Arthritis Sufferers Are Searching for the Facts. The NATIONAL ENQUIRER says: HELP IS ON THE WAY!

The more facts you know about arthritis, the better equipped you will be to deal with it. One hundred diseases are classified as arthritis. The NATIONAL ENQUIRER examines the main forms of arthritis, and outlines warning signs, methods of diagnosis, and effects on your life.

A checklist of DOs and DON'Ts for arthritis sufferers includes:

- Take a daily 20-minute bath—or shower—in warm water
- Don't use a sunlamp to heat your joints
- Do your exercises over several short periods each day—to prevent stiffened joints
- Don't allow yourself to get overweight—this puts additional pressure on the joints

LIVING WITH ARTHRITIS is not just for those who have the disease. It offers practical advice for friends and loved ones who want to offer informed support and help.

Books from The NATIONAL ENQUIRER

Conquering Stress
Famous Disasters
Living with Arthritis
UFO Report

Published by POCKET BOOKS

NATIONAL ENQUIRER

LIVING WITH ARTHRITIS

PUBLISHED BY POCKET BOOKS NEW YORK

Material in this book is based on articles previously published in The NATIONAL ENQUIRER or obtained from the Arthritis Foundation.

Another *Original* publication of POCKET BOOKS

POCKET BOOKS, a division of Simon & Schuster, Inc.
1230 Avenue of the Americas, New York, N.Y. 10020

ISBN: 0-671-52838-6

First Pocket Books printing May, 1985

10 9 8 7 6 5 4 3 2 1

Printed in the U.S.A.

CONTENTS

INTRODUCTION

Experts Reveal Simple Mental Exercise Cuts Arthritis Pain in Half! . . . Simple Gadgets Can Ease Arthritis Pain! . . . Kept Awake by Arthritis? Here Are Ten Tips to Help You Sleep . . . Woman Beats Arthritis to Become World Racquetball Champ! . . . Great News for Arthritis Victims—Clothing that's Easy to Put On.

The good news keeps pouring in. Every day new treatments, exercises, surgical procedures and practical self-help plans are being tested and improved throughout the country and the world. The research never ceases, the results are more and more promising. When all is said and done, it may some day be established that the effort to discover the causes and determine the cures for arthritis is the largest single battle ever undertaken by the medical establishment.

But until the causes and cures are finally discovered, the major focus of arthritis research and therapy must be on improving the quality of life for the arthritis patient. That means learning the dozens of different ways you can feel better, more comfortable, more nimble, more self-sufficient, more in control, more relaxed, more rested, and more optimistic.

Think for a minute about the numbers: Thirty-six million Americans suffer from arthritis. Thirty-six million men, women, and children know the pain, the fear, and discomfort of arthritis. Every thirty-three seconds brings a new case. And whether you are ten years old, sixty, or in the prime of life, you could be the next victim. You might suffer for two years or twenty. You may have pain that either comes in cycles, or is nearly constant. You may have pain and inflamation in your hip, your knees, your fingers, or even your big toe. Aspirin, heat, cold, exercise, and even sex can make you feel better. Depression, overexertion, and rainy days can make you feel worse. You may think that you have arthritis when you really don't. You may think that you have an old football injury, when you actually have arthritis. You probably think arthritis is one disease, when in fact it is one hundred.

The NATIONAL ENQUIRER has spent many years interviewing hundreds of doctors, research scientists, and other specialists in an attempt to unravel the mysteries of this disease, and to discover new and better ways for arthritis patients to beat the suffering and inconvenience connected with it. In recognition of these efforts, the Arthritis Foundation has not only awarded The NATIONAL ENQUIRER its highest honor, the Distinguished Public Service Award, the Foundation has also been an active participant in The ENQUIRER's work. It has joined forces with The NATIONAL ENQUIRER to spread the word of what can be done to help fight arthritis, and the wise counsel of the Foundation's arthritis experts is reflected in this book.

You probably have a thousand questions about arthritis, which, until now, no one has answered. Who gets arthritis? Is it chronic or does it come and go? Does surgery really work? To whom do I go for help? How do I tell the difference between a quack and a real doctor?

There are answers to all these questions—and more. Everyone can learn to live with arthritis. You have nothing to lose and everything to gain.

CHAPTER I

What Is Arthritis?

THE MISINFORMATION ABOUT ARTHRITIS CAUSES anguish and often pain. It can even lead to making your arthritis worse. Here are some of the most common myths about the disease:

MYTH: Arthritis only strikes people over forty.
FACT: Wrong, nearly every form of arthritis can strike people at any age. As many as two hundred and fifty thousand children have arthritis in the United States.

MYTH: Arthritis only affects the joints, like the hip joint or the knee.
FACT: Wrong. Other parts of the body can be affected by arthritis. For instance, *rheumatoid arthritis*, the second most common form of the disease, also may involve inflammation of the skin, lungs, heart, and other areas.

MYTH: Arthritis victims are evenly divided between men and women.

FACT: Wrong. Two thirds of all arthritis sufferers are women.

MYTH: It is better not to move around or exercise if you have arthritis.

FACT: Wrong. While in some cases, bed rest is helpful during a particularly severe attack of pain and inflammation, generally exercise is good for you. Even when you are confined to bed, passive or therapist-assisted exercise is recommended.

MYTH: Arthritis always gets worse as the victim gets older.

FACT: Wrong. While some forms of arthritis become more severe as time passes, many people suffer just one attack, which can last a few months or several years, and then never recur. Others may experience cyclical attacks, in which their arthritis may flare up for a short time and then subside, with this cycle repeating itself over the years.

MYTH: If you wake up in the morning with a stiff neck, you probably have arthritis.

FACT: Wrong. It may just be a stiff neck from tension, overexertion (too much exercise, for example), or sleeping with your neck in an awkward position. If, however, the stiffness continues for two or more weeks you should consult a doctor.

MYTH: With all the "wonder drugs" now available, aspirin is an outdated treatment for arthritis.

FACT: Wrong. Aspirin is still the most widely used drug to reduce the pain and inflammation caused by arthritis. However, because the beneficial effects of aspirin last for only a short time, repeated dosages are necessary especially for inflammation. Sometimes the newer, longer-lasting drugs are simpler to take and are the best alternative if large doses of aspirin cause side effects in the patient.

MYTH: It is impossible for the average arthritis sufferer to tell the difference between a "quack cure" and a legitimate arthritis treatment.

FACT: Wrong. It isn't really all that hard if you use some common sense. There are three warning signals that can alert you to "quackery." First: If the only evidence shown in favor of the treatment is first person statements and stories, not reports on scientific research from reputable institutions. Second: If the treatment is sold as a "cure all" for whatever ails you—from colds to cancer. Third: If it is clear that the treatment is a "get rich quick" scheme for the inventor.

MYTH: Joint replacement of a severely arthritic hip or knee can make you as good as new.

FACT: Wrong. The major goals of such surgery are to reduce the pain in that joint and to improve the function or movement within the joint. You cannot go out and play tennis or go running after such an operation.

Now you have a better understanding of just how complicated arthritis is, and how little the typical person knows about it. The only way to get to know this disease better is to start from the beginning. Let's take the word arthritis first. *Arth* means joint and *itis* means inflammation. When it comes to the world of medicine, this has got to be one of the simplest words used. Any damage, other than direct injury, inside or around any joint is called arthritis. The kind of damage that occurs determines the kind of arthritis you have. For instance, one form of arthritis has been called the "wear-and-tear" disease because it is believed by some to primarily result from the overuse or abuse of the joints. It is called *osteoarthritis.*

The kind of damage you have also determines the kind of treatment you will receive, because each form of arthritis has its own set of symptoms. This is why it is important to remember that arthritis is really a hundred different diseases all grouped under the name "arthritis." It is also important to remember that a doctor has to determine just which form of arthritis you have. Then he must prescribe the specific treatment you need. What may seem like minor pain and swelling early on could lead to the pain and crippling of severe arthritis later, if it is left untreated.

Whatever form of arthritis you have, you will be confronted with the fact that it is a chronic disease. That means it can last for a long time—from months to years or even for the length of your life. But it does not mean that you are condemned to a life of pain and suffering. It does not mean that the painful symptoms are always there for the victim of arthritis. It is typically a disease of ups and downs; sometimes the symptoms are active and severe, yet at other times, there are no symptoms at all. This back and forth rhythm is called "flare and remission." There is always hope for the arthritis sufferer, whether it is to be found in the drugs and medications of treatment, in surgery, in the natural coming and going of pain, or in the endless research being done to discover and solve the mysteries of arthritis.

What Is a Joint and How Does It Work?

To expand your understanding of arthritis, it is important to know what a joint is and how it works. A joint is any place in the body where two bones meet. For example, your thigh bone and lower leg bone meet in the middle of your leg at the kneecap. The knee is a joint. It allows the two bones, with the help of other parts of the body, to move around, to go up and down, and to bend. Without the knee we could not walk, sit, or kneel down. If you look at your hand, the point at which your fingers and your palm meet is a series of joints. Your fingers have knuckles, allowing you to form a fist or pick up a pencil. These, too, are joints.

At the joint, the ends or tips of the bones are covered by *cartilage,* a tough, elastic tissue that acts as a shock absorber. It keeps the bones from grating together. The whole joint is enclosed in a capsule that is lined by an inner skin called the *synovial membrane.* Think of the cartilage as foam-rubber padding used to pack your TV in a box so that it does not get damaged when it is shipped. And think of the capsule around the joint as one of those glass balls with snow inside that souvenir stores sell. It is made of clear glass with water inside and little white particles that look like snow floating in the water. Within the glass covering is a miniature Empire State Building or a little house with trees. When you turn the ball upside down the snow swirls around and makes the picture look like a blizzard.

Now, the capsule around the joint is like the glass ball, and the inner side of the glass is like the *synovial membrane.* The miniature building inside is the joint. The membrane releases drops of slippery fluid *(synovial fluid)* like the water in the ball, into spaces between the bones. This fluid is the "oil" in the "machinery" of the joint. It is similar to greasing a squeaky wheel or lubricating an engine. In this case, the *synovial fluid* oils the joint so it can move smoothly and easily. It also provides nutrition to keep the cartilage cells healthy.

Muscles, tendons, and ligaments are located just outside the joints. They are structures that provide support and help the bones move in the right directions. They are a little like rubber bands. If they are tight they can hold something together. When they are loose and flexible they can allow movement. Actually, *muscles* are groups of tissue which can flex and relax. They help us to move our arms and legs, our heads and backs. *Tendons* are strong, cordlike bands which connect muscles to bones. *Ligaments* are similar to tendons except that they attach bones to each other.

Fluid-filled sacs called *bursae* act as cushions to keep muscles and tendons from rubbing on bones or joints. When everything is operating properly, the machinery runs smoothly and the joint works effortlessly—and painlessly. When something goes wrong, arthritis can be the result.

Why Does a Joint Stop Working?

No one knows for certain what makes the joint machinery break down. Except for one form of arthritis, the infectious variety, scientists only have clues to the real causes of arthritic diseases.

It has been established that several human diseases are caused by unusual viruses that may live harmlessly in the body for years before becoming active and harmful. And there is a strong suspicion that a virus or something like it triggers the inflammation of some types of arthritis. But scientists do not think that everyone who has the triggering virus in his system will eventually develop arthritis. It may be that the disease only strikes people who have a particular genetic, or inherited, susceptibility to it. One clue that supports this concept is the fact that certain kinds of arthritis *(rheumatoid,* for example) have been linked with certain genetic markers. Genetic markers are like a blueprint, a guide, found in some white blood cells, which point to a tendency toward certain kinds of arthritis. Having one of these genetic markers doesn't necessarily mean you are certain to get arthritis. It may simply mean you run a higher risk of developing the disease than other people.

Immunology plays a role in producing some types of arthritis. The immune system is what enables our bodies to fight off different diseases. If a foreign substance, like a virus or bacterium, "invades" our bodies, it is the immune system which produces the "warriors" called antibodies to fight the invaders. Some scientists believe that in some arthritis victims, the immune system has gone off track and thinks that the body's *own tissue,* like the cells in our joints or the lubricating fluids, are the enemy. And, in effect, this wonderful and complex organization for fighting disease may instead create a disease itself.

Some experts in the field believe the reason some people develop *osteoarthritis* is that they were born with defective cartilage or with defects in the way their joints fit together or move. The results of such defects may not surface until the person is middle-aged or older.

Other people may develop arthritis because of an injury or because they overuse a particular joint. That "old football injury" that keeps coming back may be a form of arthritis.

Don't be discouraged that science has not found the answers to how we get arthritis. Remember that we are talking about one hundred diseases, not just one. Many of the treatments available today help control the effects of arthritis, and new drugs and programs are being developed constantly. In 1982, seventy-three million dollars were spent by the federal government to support arthritis research. The private sector has dedicated millions more in the pursuit of new remedies and an increased understanding of the disease. Some observers believe that more progress has been made in the fight against arthritis than in cancer and heart disease. But it is a tough fight, and each one of us should do his part to combat this affliction. Here is how to begin.

The Warning Signals of Arthritis

The symptoms of arthritis are as varied as the number of different kinds of arthritis. You can have aches and pains everywhere, or isolated pain in just one hand or joint. Fever and rashes, weight loss, tiredness, thickening of the skin, changes in eating habits are all signs. The Arthritis Foundation has put together a list of seven signs which may signal that you are developing arthritis. The importance of this early warning system cannot be overemphasized. Too many people ignore what their own bodies are telling them.

It's alarming and incredible, but doctors report that the average person who experiences arthritic symptoms waits four-and-a-half years before consulting a doctor. Many people not aware of the facts about arthritis postpone seeking proper medical attention. And of the people who do get help, many don't follow their treatment programs. Unfortunately, these people may later suffer permanent motion-inhibiting joint damage that could have been avoided. So whatever your arthritic symptoms may be, the first thing to do is realize that you may have a serious problem that requires immediate attention.

Seven Warning Signals

1. One or more of your joints is swollen.
2. You wake up unusually stiff in the morning.

3. You're unable to move a particular joint as easily as you once could.
4. One or more of your joints looks red and feels hot.
5. You experience unexplained weight loss, fever, or weakness, combined with joint pain.
6. Pain and tenderness recur in a particular joint.
7. Any one of these symptoms lasts for more than two weeks.

There are additional techniques that can alert you to arthritic symptoms. They include observing your hands, feet and skin.

Hand Signals

Your hands can provide some early warning signs of arthritis and may actually pinpoint what kind of arthritis you have. The early warning signs can appear before aches and pains send you to a doctor. Recognizing these signs can alert you to see a doctor, and will give you a head start in fighting arthritis and minimizing its damage to the body.

Look at Your Hands. Do You See Any of These?

• ***A hard, bony swelling*** of the middle joint of the finger and the finger joint closest to the nail. This indicates *hemachromatotic arthritis,* a very rare form of the disease which is caused by too much iron in the body.

• ***A spongy and inflamed swelling*** of the large knuckles and the middle joints of your fingers. The swelling is caused by inflammation and may feel warm to the touch. This indicates *rheumatoid arthritis,* a painful and sometimes crippling form of the disease.

• ***Tiny pits that resemble pin pricks.*** These suggest *psoriatic arthritis,* a form of the illness associated with *psoriasis,* a chronic disorder that causes red, scaly patches on the skin. Inflamed swelling of the joints of different fingers on each hand may be another warning sign of *psoriatic arthritis.* For example, your left index finger and your right ring finger may be affected at the same time. In *rheumatoid arthritis,* if swelling shows up on your right index finger, it's going to show up on your left index finger.

• ***"Clubbing" of the fingernails*** can be a warning sign of *hypertrophic pulmonary osteoarthropathy,* a rare form of arthritis that affects the lungs. Normal fingernails slope slightly downward toward the base of the nail; clubbed nails are raised and swollen.

• ***Tiny hemorrhages*** that appear underneath the fingernail as dark red spots. These could indicate *lupus,* a form of arthritis that affects the body's connective tissues and causes pain in the joints.

• ***Thickening of the fingernails*** and a change in their color from clear to opaque whiteness. These are signs of *Reiter's Syndrome,* a form of arthritis that often afflicts young men. The thickened fingernails also feel soft and chip easily.

• ***Little chalky white deposits*** next to finger joints just under the skin. These indicate *gout,* the result of too much uric acid (a chemical made by the liver) in the blood. Excess uric acid accumulates and crystallizes inside the joint where it causes pain and impedes normal function.

• *Normal wrinkles* on the back of your hands and knuckles disappear. Skin that seems drawn tight over your hands is an early sign of *scleroderma,* a form of arthritis in which skin tightens in addition to causing joint pain.

Foot Prints

The way your feet look and feel may reveal early warning signs of arthritis. "Pain and disability occur just as often—if not more frequently—in the feet of arthritis patients as they do in the hands," says Dr. John Ward, chief of the arthritis division at the University of Utah.

Some clues to the presence of *osteoarthritis* can be found in the smallest toe joints and the bunion bone, the joint at the base of your big toe. If your big toe points to the outside of your foot or if your toes are tilted upward—these may be signs of osteoarthritis.

Nearly 90 percent of people suffering from *rheumatoid arthritis* will have symptoms in their feet. They include:

- Lumps where the tip of your foot rubs against the toe of your shoe or along your Achilles' tendon at the heel.
- The bottom of your foot may have a series of what look like warts but are actually calluses.
- Your ankles may be swollen.
- Your feet may be very flat.

Skin Signals

Early warning signs can also show up on your skin. According to medical experts, here's what your skin may be telling you:

- A red, butterfly-shaped rash across the nose and cheeks may indicate *lupus,* one of the arthritic diseases that affects joints and internal organs.
- Lumps on eartips or fingertips may be a sign of *gout.*

Keep in mind that these are only warning signals that you may have arthritis. Only a doctor can make a diagnosis for certain, and you should not try to diagnose yourself.

Body Maneuvers

The following routine involves performing six body movements. They are simple maneuvers developed by the Arthritis Foundation for The NATIONAL ENQUIRER, and they provide you with an idea of how flexible and functional your joints are. They are not a means of determining whether you have arthritis, but they can indicate if you have a problem in moving your joints freely and painlessly. If you try these maneuvers repeatedly over several weeks and are unable to do them, you should consult your doctor.

The beauty of these movements is that they can be done quickly, in less than a minute. You should be able to hold each position described for five seconds. If you fail the first time, try the position again in a few weeks.

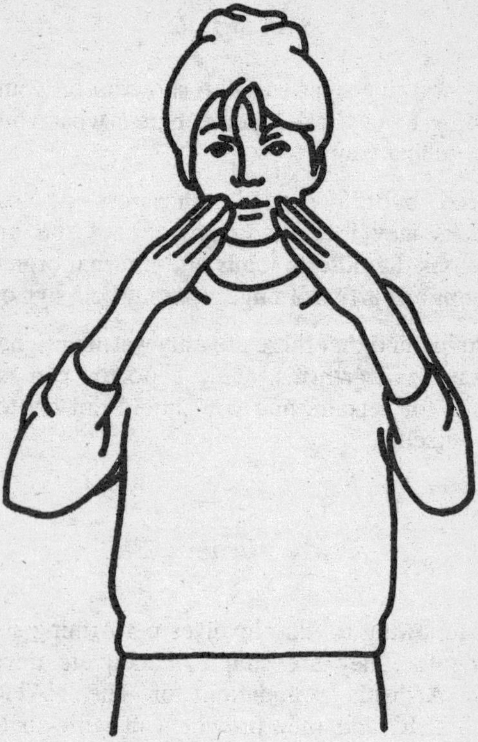

Maneuver #1: Put your hands close to, but do not touch, the corners of your mouth. Your hands should form an inverted V at roughly a forty-five-degree angle from the corners of your mouth. Your hands and arms should be in a straight line. This maneuver checks for arthritis in your elbows, shoulders, and hands.

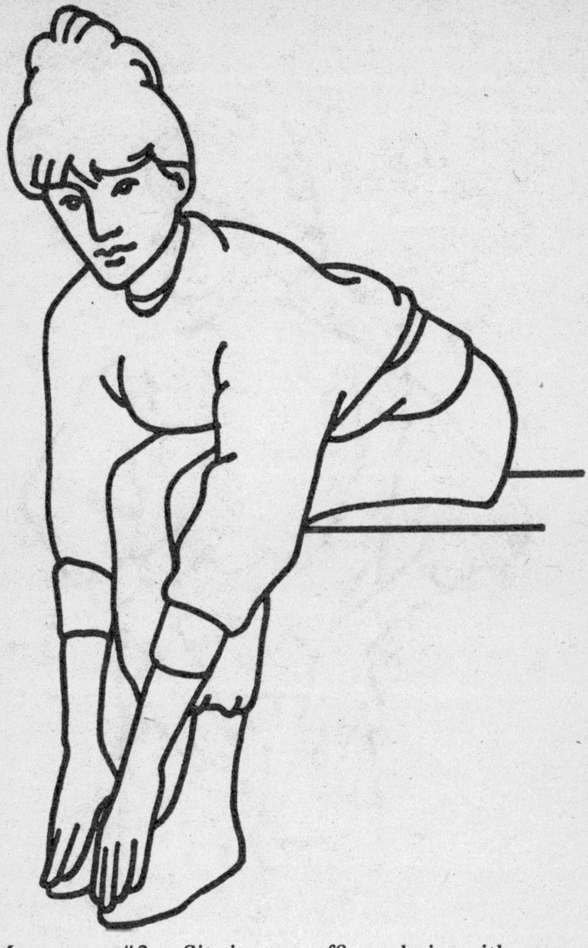

Maneuver #2: Sit in an office chair with your buttocks firmly planted at the rear of the seat. Lean over with your knees together and touch your toes, keeping your knees tucked inside your arms. This maneuver checks your knees, elbows, shoulders, back, spine, hands, and ankles.

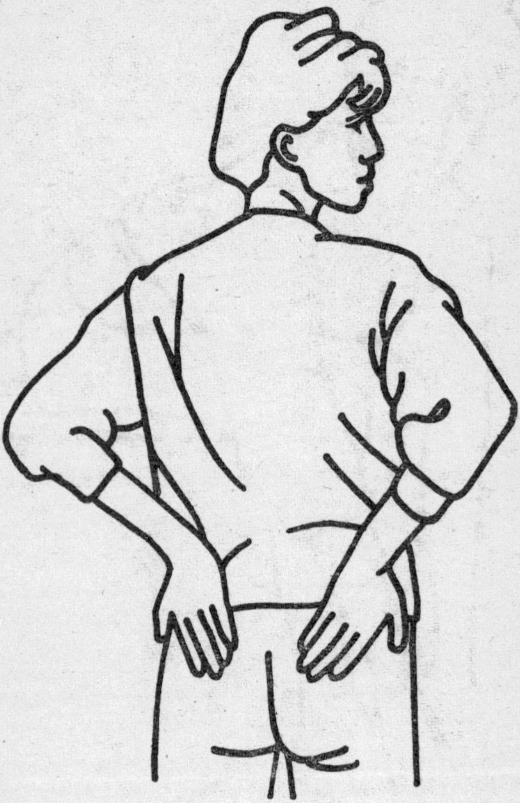

Maneuver #3: Place the flat of your hands on your upper buttocks. This maneuver checks for arthritis in your elbows, shoulders, back, neck, and hands.

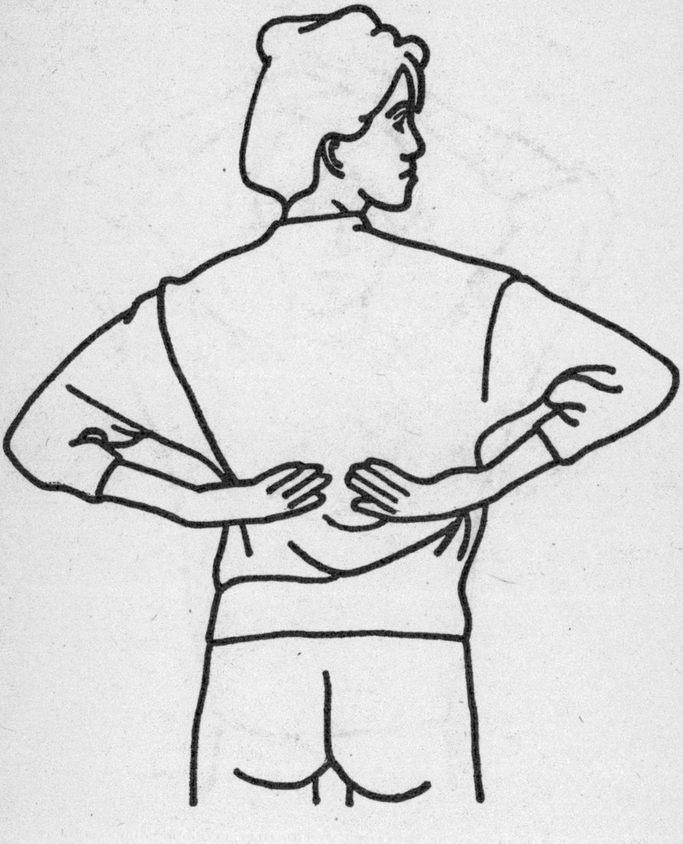

Maneuver #4: Place both hands behind your back, touching the middle of your back. This maneuver checks your elbows, shoulders, back, neck, and hands.

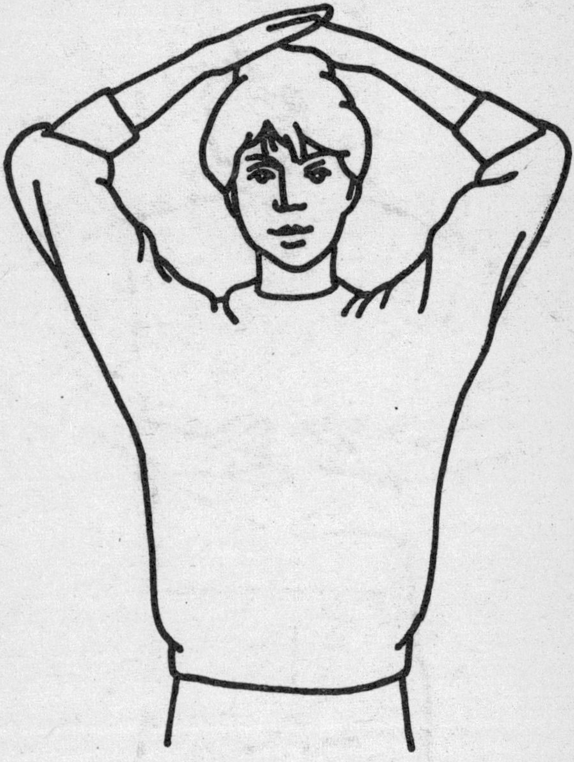

Maneuver #5: Touch the top of your head with the palms of your hands, creating a diamond shape with your hands and arms. This maneuver checks your shoulders and elbows.

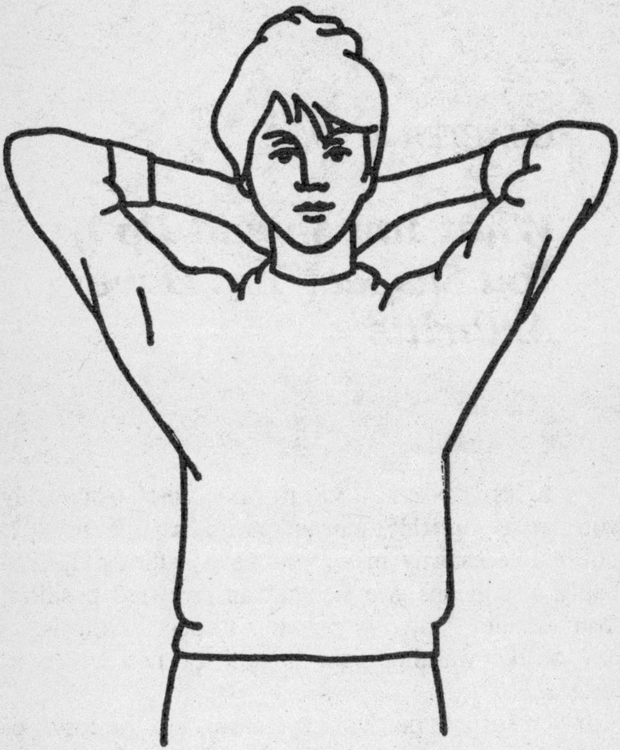

Maneuver #6: Touch the back of your neck with the palms of your hands. Your elbows, hands, and arms should form a straight line across your back at about ear level. This maneuver checks your neck, shoulders, elbows, and hands.

CHAPTER II

What You Should Do If You Suspect You Have Arthritis

FIRST, DON'T JUMP TO ANY CONCLUSIONS. IF you woke up this morning with a stiff neck it doesn't necessarily mean you have arthritis. It probably just means you slept in an awkward position. You should only begin to suspect arthritis if any of the warning signs lingers for two weeks or longer.

If you suspect that your symptoms are the result of arthritis, see your doctor. A doctor is the only one who can diagnose your condition. This doesn't mean you have to find a specialist. A family practitioner or general internist is a good person to see first. But don't put it off. Do it now.

If you don't have a family doctor because you haven't been to one lately or because your usual doctor retired, here's how to go about getting one.

Choose the Right Doctor

It's a good idea to see a family practitioner or general internist to start with because you need someone to examine the overall state of your health. These doctors have the background and experience to treat most of the common health problems that might occur in a family. Once a physician has a solid understanding of your general health, then he can identify the existence of specific ailments and recommend treatment.

Ask neighbors or co-workers for names of doctors. Do you know anybody who has arthritis and is happy with a particular doctor? Get that doctor's name, address, and phone number, too. Draw up a list of at least five doctors and check them out with the state licensing board and the American Medical Association Directory of doctors. The licensing board number can be found either in the phone book or through your telephone operator. The directory should be in your local library—just ask first. Does the doctor have a specialty? What is it? What is his or her medical training (where did he go to school)? When did he receive his medical license? Have there been any complaints filed against him—again, the licensing board can tell you this. Does the sex of the doctor make a difference to you? You should feel comfortable with the doctor you choose, male or female.

Once you have made your choice, call for an appointment. Ask what the doctor charges for a regular office visit, a checkup, a complete physical exam. Find out what costs are covered by your medical insurance plan.

you be charged for canceled appointments? Find t if the doctor is connected to a teaching hospital where medical students and young doctors train. If so, he or she may be more aware of the latest medical advances in the treatment of arthritis, or he may be involved in some of the ongoing clinical research.

When you meet the doctor, evaluate him or her as a person. Do you like this doctor? Is the doctor easy to talk to? Direct in answering your questions? Sympathetic toward you? Does the doctor treat you with concern or is he or she cold and abrupt? Do you trust this doctor?

Be Prepared

It is easy to be confused and rattled when you first meet with your doctor. You don't feel well, or you are worried and upset. It is simpler to prepare for your appointment ahead of time, when you are less agitated, than when you actually arrive in the office. You may want to write down notes to yourself to refresh your memory during your appointment. You also may wish to have a close friend or relative go to the doctor's office with you. Here are some tips on what information you should be ready to give to your doctor on your first visit.

1. *Your complete medical history,* including past illnesses; operations; vaccinations; injuries; smoking and drinking habits; any medications you are currently taking or have taken in the past few weeks; what you do for a living; how you exercise and relax; whether you're

experiencing any emotional stress; and whether your home and/or sex life are satisfactory.

2. *The current state of your health* and any abnormalities like unusual bowel movements, shortness of breath, loss of appetite, loss of weight, and so forth. Describe your aches and pains as specifically as you can. Do you ache all over, or only in one spot? Is it a dull, throbbing pain or is it sharp and stabbing? Does the pain come and go, or is it constant? Are you in more pain in the morning than at night?

3. *Your family's general medical history* is important, too. Some forms of arthritis may be hereditary. Does anyone in your family (mother, grandfather, uncle, niece) have arthritis or any other serious disease? There may be clues in this information to your condition which are hidden from you, but are relevant to your doctor's diagnosis.

The Physical Examination and the Most Common Tests

After the doctor gets a record of your medical history and listens to your current health concerns, a general practitioner will probably perform a complete physical examination and include several well-known tests. It is the doctor's responsibility to read and analyze the results of any test. But today, most of us want to be better informed about just what the doctor is doing and why. An examining room can be a cold and frightening place and it can reassure you to know what is going on.

One test is a *complete blood count* (CBC) which determines:

1. The number of *white blood cells.* These cells multiply rapidly when infections and inflammation are present in your body.

2. The *hemoglobin count.* Hemoglobin is a protein found in the *red blood cells.* It contains the mineral iron and carries oxygen to every part of your body.

3. The *hematocrit* count. This measures the percentage of red blood cells in your blood.

4. The number of *platelets.* These are tiny elements in the blood which help your blood to clot (without them a simple cut could make us bleed to death).

The doctor may also measure your *blood sedimentation* (SED) rate by measuring the speed at which red cells settle in unclotted blood. Red cells settle faster than normal in patients with inflammation and other disorders. The results of the SED rate test can be used as a guide to the severity of a disease and to your response to drug therapy.

In addition, the doctor can check your blood for the presence of *C-Reactive Protein* (CRP), a protein which is more abundant during inflammation or tissue destruction. This test is also used as a guide to what the disease is doing (getting worse or getting better), and how it is responding to drugs.

Most physical examinations include *urine analyses.* There are two main types: 1) A routine *urinalysis* to detect substances not normally present in the urine, such as sugar, proteins, bacteria, and blood; 2) A *urine culture* to detect the type and quantity of bacteria present in the urine. Once this has been established, the doctor can prescribe the appropriate antibiotic. Similar cultures can be made of blood and other body fluids (e.g. mucus) as well as tissue culture of body openings (e.g. mouth) and organs if there is a possibility of infection.

The doctor may order a *chemistry survey,* also called SMA6, SMA12, SMAC. This is a group of tests performed on a single sample of blood, which monitor substances that are normally present in blood but may be abnormally high or low in number because of the presence of a disease or the use of a specific treatment. A chemistry survey can analyze your body's nutritional health, kidney function, hormonal balance, liver and muscle function, the condition of your bones, levels of cholesterol and other fats (which can contribute to coronary disease), glucose levels, and the presence of diabetes.

The doctor might also perform a complete examination of your ears, nose, throat, neck, chest, and abdomen to check for any abnormalities or sensitivities.

Some Specialized Arthritis Tests

If your doctor has diagnosed arthritis, he will want to determine which form of the disease you have. The tests described below can help in five important ways. They can: (1) Help to confirm a diagnosis of which type of arthritis is present; (2) Determine how the arthritis affects, or is affected by, your general health; (3) Discover the severity of your disease; and (4) Monitor the response of the disease to therapy. Remember that negative test results do not eliminate the possibility that a particular disease exists—they just help your doctor make an informal diagnosis.

A procedure called the *latex test* detects the presence of something called the *rheumatoid factor.* Although levels of this factor usually indicate *rheumatoid arthri-*

tis, a negative latex test does not necessarily mean that you definitely do not have this disease. Similarly, latex test results in the low positive range don't always mean that you do have rheumatoid arthritis.

The *Antinuclear Antibodies* (ANA) test detects the presence of proteins that are usually absent in the general population. People suffering from any form of arthritis which affects their whole body tend to have high levels of these specific proteins.

Other Tests

These general tests are often used as part of the diagnostic procedure.

X-Ray—An X-ray reveals changes that may have taken place in bone, cartilage or other structures as a result of arthritis. Sometimes special liquid dyes are injected into the patient to highlight the areas being examined.

Bone Scan—A small amount of radioactive material injected into a patient's vein is used in this test to detect inflammation and is often helpful when an X-ray does not show any abnormality.

Salicylate Level—Salicylate is the active ingredient in aspirin and can be very effective in the treatment of arthritis when it is taken in the proper amounts. This test measures the concentration of salicylate in the blood so that the dosage can be adjusted if necessary.

Biopsy—This test enables a doctor to examine tissue from an organ or muscle by inserting a hollow needle into the area and drawing out a tiny piece of the tissue.

Tapping—Excess fluid that can accumulate around an affected joint is sometimes drawn off using a hollow needle.

While some of these tests may be uncomfortable, the information they provide can be critically important to a correct diagnosis and treatment.

After the Visit to Your Doctor

After you've seen the doctor, evaluate how the appointment went. Did the doctor rush you? Did he listen carefully to what you told him? Did he take notes as you were talking? Did he give you any test without a *clear* explanation? Were his descriptions of any problems you might have and the treatment he prescribed straightforward and understandable? Did the doctor answer your questions? Don't be intimidated. You have the right to understand what is wrong with you. Make sure you ask your doctor to explain what he is doing in simple terms.

Remember that a second opinion can be valuable, especially when you're trying to establish whether you have something as serious as arthritis. You have every right to go to another doctor to see whether he confirms what your first physician said and the treatment he prescribed. Good health and the proper medical care are essential to the quality of your life. You are the only one who can judge whether you are receiving the correct care. And you have the right to make sure that you do.

If for some reason you feel you won't be able to follow the doctor's advice and prescribed treatment, be sure to speak up. For example, if your doctor tells you to lose some weight and you know that is a very hard thing for you to do, then the doctor should know that.

This way the doctor can adjust his advice to help you achieve the same goal with less stress and strain. If you can't take a medication your doctor prescribes because it costs too much, the doctor may be able to find a less expensive substitute. But first you have to tell him. If you do fall off a treatment plan, don't just say "the heck with it." Tell your doctor at once—he may be able to help you over the stumbling block or find an alternative method.

The Arthritis Specialists

If your general practitioner has diagnosed arthritis you may want to seek out a specialist. Ask your doctor to recommend one. Or contact your local chapter of the Arthritis Foundation (see Appendix) and find out if they have any recommendations for specialists near you. The kinds of "specialists" you can see about arthritis range from highly regarded professionals who are sanctioned by the American Medical Association and the Arthritis Foundation to quacks. You will want to be very careful.

More than likely, the kind of specialist you'll want is a *rheumatologist,* a doctor who specializes in treating arthritis patients. There are only 3,000 rheumatologists in the U.S. and just 5 percent of arthritis sufferers go to them. Most rheumatologists are also internists, which means they have been trained in general adult health care.

You might choose to consult a chiropractor. Chiropractic healing is based on the theory that pain and discomfort are caused by the impaired functioning of the nerves related to the spinal column. Through manual manipulation of different parts of the body, a chiropractor aims to give you relief from aches and pains. If you choose a chiropractor, you should know that the American Medical Association does not endorse the presence of chiropractors in the medical field because a chiropractor earns his degree from a chiropractic, rather than a medical, school. His four years of training include basic anatomy, physiology, biochemistry, microbiology, pathology, and the interpretation of X-ray films.

You should not visit a chiropractor until you know from your doctor that you do not have some serious form of arthritis that needs medical treatment.

People with lower back pains, including arthritis patients, may find relief from a physical therapist. A study conducted at the University of Washington showed that "patients with lower back pain who were treated by physical therapists expressed significantly greater relief than those who were treated by internal medicine specialists," says Dr. Overman of the Arthritis Resource Center in Seattle.

Physical therapists often give their patients an exercise program to follow, teach them how to correct their posture and modify their activities, and teach them how to protect the painful area of the lower back to prevent additional injury.

Many family doctors are likely to prescribe a week's bed rest, and muscle relaxants or painkillers, which treat the symptoms but not necessarily the ailment. Some will even include simple exercises along with medicine and rest.

Dr. Frederic McDuffie, Senior Vice President of Medical Affairs for the Arthritis Foundation, says:

"While it is extremely important that a patient see a family doctor or internist first, it is true that physical therapists can offer relief to arthritis sufferers who have pain in the lower back."

Physical therapists should not be a replacement for doctors if you have arthritic symptoms, but they might prove to be helpful in relieving pain in conjunction with your other treatment. Your doctor and therapist should work together in developing your treatment program.

The Arthritis Team

There are arthritis clinics and special centers where rheumatologists work with a team of other health professionals to provide total care for the victims of arthritis. In addition to a rheumatologist, an arthritis team will almost certainly have a nurse who has received special training in rheumatology.

Other members of an arthritis team may also include:

- A physical therapist who provides training in special exercises and the use of different kinds of heat treatment to relieve arthritis pain.
- An occupational therapist who provides advice about necessary changes in daily activities, suggests recreational activities, and helps the patient adjust to therapy.
- A physiatrist who is a doctor specializing in physical therapy and medicine, and is involved in the evaluation and non-surgical treatment of deformities that may result from arthritis.
- An orthopedist who is a surgeon and will be involved if you need surgery.

- A medical social worker who counsels the patient regarding his personal, family, or financial problems, and about the emotional aspects of illness.
- A psychologist who counsels the patient on emotional difficulties and is also trained to do psychological testing.
- A psychiatrist who is a medical doctor specializing in mental health and who treats emotional problems.
- A pharmacist who can answer questions about the medication you may be taking, including information about which brands are cheapest and the possible side effects you may experience.
- A dietician who can teach you about good nutrition and can assist in planning your meals.
- An opthalmologist or eye doctor who will check for signs of eye problems and treat eye disease.

CHAPTER III

The Two Most Common Forms of Arthritis

OF THE 109 DIFFERENT DISEASES THAT ARE grouped under the label "arthritis," the following two are the most prevalent by far. A description of each will give you a general idea of the various complications that can cause arthritic pain.

Osteoarthritis

Osteoarthritis is perhaps man's oldest and most widespread disease. Beginning at least with the dinosaurs, almost every animal that can walk has been susceptible to this form of arthritis. It's certain that the majority of people over the age of sixty suffer from *osteoarthritis* of some joints, at least to a slight degree. Medical treatment isn't necessary unless the condition causes pain or other symptoms.

In simple terms, *osteoarthritis* is a disease of the joints that involves a breakdown of cartilage and other tissues which enable a joint to operate smoothly. It usually affects individual joints like one knee or hip. The damage is confined to the joint and surrounding tissues. There is little or no inflammation, but pain, stiffness, and limited function of the affected joint do occur.

Osteoarthritis is called the "wear and tear" arthritis by some experts because they believe it is the result of a lifetime of demands being placed on a joint. Others disagree with this description and insist that it is abnormal stress on a joint which eventually injures it. These experts cite obesity, bones that aren't lined up correctly, certain jobs which stress the joints, bad posture, and injuries as the causes. There are even some doctors and researchers who think *osteoarthritis* develops for all of these reasons and add heredity as well.

Who Has Osteoarthritis?

Sixteen million people in the United States have *osteoarthritis* severe enough to cause painful problems. And another thirty million people might very well show evidence of the disease on X-rays but experience no painful symptoms. Ninety-seven percent of everyone over the age of sixty have some symptoms of *osteoarthritis* even if they can't see or feel them. The older you are, the more likely you are to have some recognizable evidence of this disease. If you're a woman, you have twice as much chance of getting the disease as a man. Constant and excessive wear and tear on the joints can speed the process that results in *osteoarthritis.*

Does Osteoarthritis Have Other Names?

Yes, several. *Osteoarthritis* may also be labeled "degenerative joint disease." Some doctors also call it *arthrosis, osteoarthrosis,* and *hypertrophic arthritis.*

What Are the Effects of Osteoarthritis?

The first noticeable effect is a softening, pitting, and fraying of the cartilage surface which cushions the joint. The joint tissue loses its elasticity and becomes susceptible to further damage caused by stress.

As the disease progresses, whole sections of cartilage may be worn away completely, leaving only smooth bone ends exposed to each other. Without the gliding, slippery surfaces of normal cartilage to help, it may become painful to move the joint.

As the cartilage continues to disintegrate, the joint begins to lose its normal shape, the underlying bone ends become thickened, and bony spurs may form where the ligaments are attached. Cysts may form in the bone near the joint, and fragments of bone or cartilage may break loose within the joint.

In severe *osteoarthritis,* the normal shape and mechanical structure of the joint are destroyed.

Where Does Osteoarthritis Occur?

Although this disease can strike any of your joints, certain joints are more prone to it than others. Normally it attacks one joint at a time and, except in the fingers, seldom moves from one joint to another. The most commonly involved joints are the fingers and those that bear weight, such as your spine, hips, and knees.

The condition seldom affects the base of the fingers, the wrists, the elbows, shoulders, or ankles, except when these joints have been injured, are diseased, or are subjected to repeated strains as might occur in athletics or physically demanding occupations such as ballet dancing.

Is There More Than One Kind of Osteoarthritis?

Doctors tend to separate the disease into two kinds: primary and secondary. When the disease seems to start by itself, without any apparent injury or other triggering event, it is called *primary osteoarthritis.* When the disease seems to result from abnormal physical stress or injury, it is called *secondary osteoarthritis.* The term refers to the fact the condition is "secondary" to, or the result of, stress or strain.

There are several general differences between the two aspects of the disease. *Primary osteoarthritis* is more of an overall condition. It occurs mostly in women, and usually affects small joints, particularly those in the fingers and hands. It happens somewhat early in life, occasionally striking people in their late thirties and early forties, and seems to be more common in some families than in others.

Secondary osteoarthritis tends to affect the larger joints although it can strike small joints which are exposed to excessive stress and strain. As a rule, it occurs late in life, but it can come along earlier if a particular joint has been injured.

What Triggers Osteoarthritis?

Often, the pattern in which joints are affected can be linked to a person's job. A job that requires standing for long periods will put strain on the knees and ankles. Constant use of the hands, such as in typing, may create problems in the wrists and fingers. Of course, sports that involve repeated and often abnormal stress on joints can also be a factor in the development of *osteoarthritis*. So can obesity, injuries, and bad posture.

Dr. George Ehrlich, formerly Chief Rheumatologist at the Albert Einstein Medical Center in Philadelphia, believes that most runners will have knee and, perhaps, hip problems in the future. Medical evidence, he says, indicates that 70 to 80 percent of all runners experience painful joints at the very least.

Dr. Stanford H. Roth, director of the Phoenix Arthritis Center in Arizona, said that he and other medical specialists have discussed the growing problem of running-related arthritis but they do not know how to solve it. "We are encountering a large number of young people who are jogging today and laying the groundwork for some possible arthritic conditions in the future," Roth says.

What Are the Symptoms of Osteoarthritis?

Pain is a common symptom of *osteoarthritis*. Most patients experience only minor aching and soreness, particularly when they try to move certain joints. Some patients have constant, nagging pain which persists even at rest. The pain of *osteoarthritis* may be confined to the joint or it may spread to the surrounding area. In some rare instances, you may feel pain quite a distance away from the joint. This is called "referred pain." For example, an osteoarthritic hip may produce pain in the region of the knees.

Another major symptom is *loss of mobility.* If you find yourself unable to perform routine tasks such as turning a doorknob or writing a note without pain or discomfort, then you may have osteoarthritic problems.

A third symptom is difficulty in moving a joint. If it seems to take more energy to move a joint, this may be a related symptom of *osteoarthritis.*

What Causes the Bony Knobs on Fingers?

These are *Heberden's nodes.* They are bony enlargements of the end joints of the fingers that are most often seen in *primary osteoarthritis* in women, sometimes appearing as early as age forty. There is a tendency for *Heberden's nodes* to run in families. Similar enlargements of the middle joints on the fingers are called *Bouchard's nodes.* Both nodes may also result from a stress injury to the finger such as "bowler's finger" or "baseball finger."

Typical *Heberden's nodes* are multiple, first appearing on one finger and then spreading to others. They may be painless, or they can appear suddenly with redness, swelling, tenderness, and aching. Patients with *Heberden's nodes* may complain of numbness and tingling of the fingertips and clumsiness of the hands.

Although *Heberden's nodes* can be painful and unsightly, they seldom severely impair the use of your hands. Crippling is not likely to occur.

What Tests Are Used to Diagnose Osteoarthritis?

Doctors agree that the most valuable aid in diagnosing *osteoarthritis* is a series of X-rays. These show the physician the typical changes in joint structure that must be present in order to diagnose *osteoarthritis.*

Sometimes blood counts are performed when the patient is first examined, and again at frequent intervals when certain treatments and medications have been prescribed. Occasionally, a detailed analysis of joint fluid *(synovial fluid)* may be necessary, because the presence of this fluid in excess amounts, sometimes called "water-on-the-joint," causes the joint (usually the knee) to swell. The excess fluid can be removed quite easily by inserting a needle into the joint and withdrawing the fluid through the needle.

What Can Be Done for Osteoarthritis?

While *osteoarthritis* is not a disease that, at this time, can be cured, its symptoms can be alleviated, and impaired joint function can be improved. In these days of medical wonders and astonishing scientific advances, many people think there ought to be a drug, a pill, or an injection that will cure anything that ails them. But since *osteoarthritis* is mainly due to mechanical factors, it is not likely that any drug will ever be found to cure it.

Osteoarthritis is one of a number of chronic diseases for which treatment involves doing a number of things instead of just one or two. Your treatment for *osteoarthritis* will probably involve the following steps:

- Controlling pain and discomfort with drugs.
- Protecting the joints from stresses and strains.
- Correcting faulty joint mechanisms.
- Maintaining an exercise schedule and a hearty diet.

The Show Must Go On

Did you know that Melvyn Douglas had arthritis? Or Katharine Hepburn? Or John Carradine, Raymond Massey, James Garner, Joan Blondell and Henry Fonda? They also have other things in common—they all are or were actors, well-known stars of stage and screen, and heroes. Heroes and heroines because they never gave into their arthritis. They have taken their pain and suffering and varying degrees of disability, looked them straight in the face and said: "Nothing will stop me, not even you!"

Despite what we may think of Hollywood stars—how pampered they are, and how rich and spoiled—we now know that these stars have fought on when they could easily have given in. They could have retired with the money they had earned in their illustrious careers—but they didn't.

Henry Fonda's courageous battle is typical of all these heroes. Tormented by arthritis in his hip, legendary trooper Henry Fonda battled searing pain and the pleas of doctors, family, and friends that he stop working for a while—because he wanted the show to go on.

His ordeal began in March of 1979, in Los Angeles, when he tripped during a performance of the play *First Monday in October*. Fonda recalled he had felt pain for some time. "I just didn't wince on stage," he said. "Every now and then I would limp, but not too much."

Fonda suffered in silence while the play ended its West Coast run and moved on to Chicago. The play opened, and he performed without a hitch until one morning he stretched out in bed and heard a snap in his left leg. The pain increased sharply and became unbearable. It reached the point where he had to be carried out and raced to a hospital that afternoon.

Chicago doctors diagnosed his condition as inflammation from arthritis, but Fonda insisted that the show had to go on even if he had to use crutches. As his wife Shirlee revealed later, "His drive for the theater is so strong that he wanted to defy the orders of the doctors. To him theater comes first. But he has to start thinking about himself, because he never does."

Fonda was convinced finally that he should stay in bed. Later, when he returned to California, he had surgery on his hip. It was at that time the doctors discovered cancerous cells in his prostate.

Fonda's old-time friend and fellow veteran of the screen and stage, Jimmy Stewart, summed it all up when he said, "There's absolutely nothing that can keep him down. He never complains. He doesn't want to burden his family or friends with his pain. He is an old trooper."

Henry Fonda overcame his medical problems and went back to work, performing right up until the time he died.

Rheumatoid Arthritis

Throughout the years, *rheumatoid arthritis* (RA) has been one of medical science's most elusive puzzles. Of the more than one hundred forms of arthritis, RA is the most serious, the most painful, and the most potentially crippling. It can affect the whole body, causing disease and inflammation in the lungs, skin, blood vessels, muscles, heart, and even the eyes.

RA has been medically identified for about two hundred years, indicating that it probably represents a fairly recent disease in man.

What Is Rheumatoid Arthritis?

Rheumatoid arthritis is more than just arthritis. Many doctors refer to it as the "rheumatoid disease" to emphasize its widespread effects on the body. The term "rheum" describes the stiffness, body aches, and fatigue that often accompany the disease. Patients with RA often say they feel like they have a virus. They may be right.

No one knows the specific cause of RA. Physicians and researchers believe that though RA is not inherited, a genetic factor may lead to lowered disease resistance. This susceptibility may be triggered later in life by a virus. This theoretical virus can cause perplexing disturbances in the body's *immune system.* One of the most active areas of research into RA concerns the definite identification of this gene and its connection to possible viral infection.

The *immune system* is the defense mechanism your body uses to fight off disease. When it's working properly, your *immune system* attacks "invaders" (viruses and bacteria) from outside the body. But in *rheumatoid arthritis,* your immune system malfunctions and attacks perfectly normal tissues and fluids. This war within the body is called an *autoimmune reaction,* and the greatest destruction occurs in the joints.

Who Has RA?

About two million people definitely have RA in the United States and another five million people probably have it. Three of every four victims of RA are women. The disease usually sets in after the age of twenty and before sixty, but it can begin as early as infancy or as late as age ninety.

What Are the Effects of RA?

Its effects are many and have a significant impact on your body. The disease can start in one or more joints without warning. The same joint is usually involved on both sides of the body—if you've got it in the right hand, chances are you also have it in the left hand (though it is usually worse in the right, if you are right-handed). RA tends to affect particular joints, especially those in the feet, arms, hips, hands, and legs. In most cases several joints become involved, particularly those of the hands and feet.

When a joint is struck by RA, its inner workings begin to deteriorate. The *synovial membrane* thickens and swelling increases. The membrane grows like a tongue between the two layers of cartilage of the two bones forming a joint. This tongue invades the cartilage and eventually the bone underneath, destroying it.

The joint becomes inflamed. It swells. It gets hot. It turns red. And it causes pain, which usually gets worse with movement. The joint may be least painful in a partially bent position because the pressure inside an inflamed joint decreases in such a position.

But if you don't move a painful joint, it can quickly become stiff, and the muscles surrounding it can become useless. This leads, over a prolonged period, to the loss of motion and function, weakness and more pain. You can ease the pain by learning to warm up the joint through gentle exercises that slowly move the joints through their entire range-of-motion (see p. 83). Today, the possibility of severe crippling is less than ever before with continued therapy.

Other effects of RA are weakness and fatigue, loss of appetite, and loss of weight. Many patients have cold, sweaty hands and feet. Patients with RA may also experience inflammation of the eyes, inflammation of the area around the lungs, and general anemia, which is a reduction of the oxygen-carrying cells in the blood.

In addition, RA sufferers may have lumps or nodules under the skin. These are called *rheumatoid nodules* and can range from the size of a pea to the size of a mothball.

In summary, here's a checklist of specific symptoms of RA:

- Swelling and pain in one or more joints that last at least six weeks.
- Both sides of the body are affected.
- The wrists and knuckles are almost always involved.
- General fatigue, weakness, and loss of weight and appetite.

Only a combination of several of these symptoms should lead you to suspect RA. Fatigue and weakness might be a sign of lack of sleep. A swollen joint may be the result of a strain, and nothing more. And even if you do suffer from these symptoms, it's up to your doctor to officially make a diagnosis of *rheumatoid arthritis*.

Does RA Ever Go Away?

Yes and no. It is typically a disease of ups and downs—flares and remissions. It's not uncommon for the symptoms to lessen significantly for periods of weeks, months, or even years. In at least one out of every five cases, the symptoms seem to disappear completely. But they can return later, with even greater force than before. You may feel as though your RA has disappeared, but after an examination your doctor may still find evidence of the disease. It is still present but in remission, as if it were asleep.

The symptoms' duration has been broken down into three patterns by doctors. The first (and best) pattern consists of a brief illness that lasts a few months or less and leaves no disability; this pattern is called *monocyclic.* The second pattern involves periods of illness separated by periods of well-being; this pattern is called *polycyclic* and usually results in little serious physical impairment. The third, the *chronic* pattern, lasts a number of years, sometimes for life. Serious crippling is not the inevitable outcome of this form of the disease. It is likely that early and continuous treatment could have prevented the severe deformity and crippling you may have seen in some people. That's why it's essential that you consult a doctor as soon as you suspect any form of arthritis.

How Does a Doctor Diagnose RA?

A doctor should carefully review all of your health complaints, including symptoms or injuries you may have experienced years ago. He should perform a general examination and pay special attention to the joints, noting signs of inflammation, loss of movement, or other abnormalities. To identify the presence of RA or another form of arthritis, the doctor will perform several of the blood tests we outlined earlier, such as tests for the *rheumatoid factor.* These tests are called by several names, such as *latex test, sheep cell test,* and *bentonite test.* They are not always conclusive, but they can be helpful in confirming a diagnosis.

The *sedimentation rate test,* also used in diagnosing *osteoarthritis,* can be useful here. Unlike people with *osteoarthritis,* those with *rheumatoid arthritis* have fast sedimentation rates.

Analysis of joint fluid can help a doctor determine which type of arthritis is present. X-rays are useful but not necessarily conclusive in detecting RA. A doctor may request X-rays of specific joints periodically to determine how the disease is progressing.

There will be a discussion of other arthritis-related diseases later in the book. One affects children exclusively, others are rare but dangerous, and one is infectious. For the moment, let's take a look at treatments. It is difficult enough to deal with the fact that you may have arthritis, but if you don't know the full range of remedies and treatments, arthritis can sound more frightening than it should. And, if you know for sure that you do have the disease, it will be encouraging and educational to have a complete review of what methods are being used to deal with arthritis. Perhaps you may even want to talk to your doctor about some of these treatments and whether they can help you.

CHAPTER IV

Arthritis Treatments: Drugs

WHILE TREATMENTS FOR THE SYMPTOMS OF ARthritis can include exercise, surgery, and experimental therapies, drugs are also an effective and crucial ingredient in dealing with these diseases. There are numerous safety factors involved in taking drugs, having prescriptive drugs in your home, and recognizing and coping with side effects. This chapter deals with all these areas and gives you some insights into what research is being done in this field.

An effective program of drug therapy for arthritis should be tailored for your personal needs. As you have seen, there are many forms of arthritis and each affects its victims differently. Also, every patient has a unique reaction to any given medication. Your doctor should decide which medications are appropriate for you and your specific ailment.

Guidelines for Taking Drugs

Make sure you tell your doctor about any other drugs you're taking now or have taken in the past two weeks. Some drugs can react badly in your body when they are combined and you must be very careful to take only the drugs your doctor has specifically prescribed for you. If you are taking medicines for other ailments or illnesses your doctor has to be made aware of what they are and why you are taking them.

- ***Keep all drugs out of reach of children.*** Drugs can easily pass for candy and a child can die from taking even a small dosage mistakenly.
- ***Follow your doctor's instructions carefully.*** You should know what the medication is, how much to take, how often to take it, and how long to continue taking it. Someone you know may be taking the same drug but of a different strength or with different instructions; your instructions have been tailored to your needs.
- ***Take your medicine exactly as your doctor prescribes.*** Never change the dosage on your own. If one pill is good for you, two are not necessarily better.
- ***Take all arthritis medication with food unless otherwise directed.*** Many arthritis drugs can irritate the stomach lining. The "sandwich technique" (eat a little food, take your medication, eat a little more food) can help prevent irritation.
- ***Keep each medication separate*** in a labeled container. Mixing medications can lead to harmful chemical interactions—or worse, you may take the wrong drug by mistake.

• ***Give your medication time to work.*** Don't grow impatient if you don't see immediate results—ask your doctor when you might reasonably expect to see some improvement in your condition.

• ***Ask your pharmacist for non-childproof containers.*** Many arthritis patients have difficulty opening those push, twist, and pull containers.

• ***Always bring whatever medications you're taking with you*** when you visit your doctor, and have them near the phone if you're going to call your doctor.

• ***Always report any side effects*** or unusual reactions such as rashes, nausea, fever, vomiting, headaches, or anything else abnormal to your doctor.

• ***Above all, be honest with your doctor.*** If you haven't been taking your medication as prescribed, tell your doctor, otherwise he may make changes in your treatment which could be harmful.

• ***Never stop taking medication*** until or unless your doctor tells you to.

• ***Don't drive or operate heavy machinery if you feel drowsy*** from your medication. Your doctor can tell you if any of the medications he prescribes are likely to make you drowsy.

• ***Don't let your medication run out*** before ordering more refills. Stopping a steady flow of medication might cause your arthritis to flare.

• ***Don't take old medication.*** Outdated medicines can be ineffective or even dangerous.

• ***And lastly, don't expect medication to provide total relief*** all by itself. A combination of drugs, exercise, joint protection, weight control, and regular medical examinations are essential to achieve adequate control of arthritic diseases.

How to Make the Best Use of Your Medication

Though it's essential to follow your doctor's prescription concerning the dose and frequency of your aspirin intake, you can minimize the pain of *rheumatoid* and *osteoarthritis* by matching the time you take medication with the times your arthritis predictably flares up. What's more, this simple practice will also reduce the risk of side effects.

Rheumatoid arthritis symptoms—such as pain, inflammation, and swelling—are more intense at certain times of the day than at others. These symptoms tend to reach a peak between 2 and 4 A.M. at night and fall to their lowest level about 4 in the afternoon.

Since short-acting medications—such as aspirin, Motrin, and Indocin—take roughly two hours to reach their peak effectiveness, you should take them about two hours in advance of your peak period of pain. That way, the drug will reach its own maximum activity at the same time your pain is at its maximum level.

Amazingly, by merely adjusting the time you take your arthritis medication you can actually reduce your rheumatoid arthritis symptoms with less medicine and, at the same time, diminish the risk of side effects.

Because everyone's periods of pain are different, you should keep a written record of your own for a few days and then show it to your doctor so he can help you develop a schedule for taking your drugs most effectively.

It is important to know, however, that this system works only with short-acting drugs. It doesn't apply to long-lasting arthritis medication such as gold and pencillamine.

Aspirin, the Wonder Drug

It may come as a surprise to learn that aspirin really is the most widely used drug in the treatment of arthritis. Furthermore, a recent scientific study reveals that aspirin is the most effective pain reliever for controlling mild to moderate arthritis pain. [*Note:* Everyone responds differently to medication. Keep in mind that even though aspirin might be the most effective medicine, an individual's body chemistry and the kind of arthritis he has may mean that another medication will be more effective for him in controlling his symptoms.]

The study, conducted by Dr. Joe Hardin, Jr., a rheumatologist and associate professor of internal medicine at the University of South Alabama College of Medicine, tested the five most commonly used drugs for the treatment of arthritis. Aspirin was found to give the most effective relief.

"We found aspirin to be the superior agent in patients with mild to moderate pain," Dr. Hardin said. "This is true for both *osteo-* and *rheumatoid arthritis.*"

If you are told to take aspirin, your doctor will tell you how much to take, and when to take it. Perhaps you can't tolerate as much aspirin as someone else can without experiencing side effects. You may even be one of the few people who can't take aspirin at all. In that case, your doctor will prescribe alternatives to aspirin.

Aspirin is a member of the *salicylate family*. Each member of this group reduces the effects of inflammation, including pain, swelling, redness, and heat. The word *salicylate* refers to the active ingredient in aspirin and other drugs. Aspirin is the most familiar of the *salicylates*.

Small amounts of *salicylates* relieve headaches, mild pain and fever. Larger dosages taken regularly over a period of time relieve some of the symptoms associated with the inflammation of arthritis. Still, larger amounts can cause poisoning, which can be mild or severe. Your physician should always supervise any changes or adjustments in how much medicine you take.

Aspirin and other salicylates belong to a group of drugs called *non-steroidal anti-inflammatory drugs* (or NSAIDs). All NSAIDs have the ability to reduce the effects of inflammation as their name implies, yet each individual arthritis sufferer reacts differently to these drugs. Some find great relief and others respond less favorably to NSAIDs. They are not related to steroid drugs which represent a different group of anti-inflammatory drugs discussed later in this chapter (see p. 72). The NSAIDs appear to work by blocking the action of natural chemicals in the body that cause some of the pain and inflammation of arthritis.

Although aspirin is similar to other NSAIDs in its effect on arthritis, it does have one big advantage: it costs a lot less than the others. Since arthritis patients usually have to take medication for many months, aspirin's relatively low cost is often a major factor in its selection as part of a prescribed drug therapy.

How Much Aspirin Should I Take?

When you are in pain it is difficult to deny yourself medicine which can make you feel better. But here you have to be strong and you have to learn to trust your doctor, otherwise you can harm or even kill yourself. Only your doctor can determine how much aspirin you need to take to effectively treat the symptoms of your disease, and how much your body can tolerate.

You can make a serious mistake if you try to figure out your own medication dosages and schedule. Each person's body handles aspirin in a different way. And each person's arthritic symptoms react differently to aspirin or any medication. A daily dose that's just right for one person may be too small for another, and cause poisoning in a third. Your doctor has the knowledge and experience needed to determine the proper dose for you.

If you need intensive treatment with aspirin, your doctor will ask you to alert him to any side effects you experience, and he may periodically check the level of *salicylate* in your blood. Based on this information he will be able to adjust the dosage so that it is most effective for you. When the proper amount you need and can tolerate without dangerous side effects has been determined, you must take it regularly: A certain blood level of aspirin must be maintained to produce the desired effects. Therefore, the benefits of aspirin may be lost if it is not taken exactly as prescribed.

Read the Label

Different brands of aspirin contain varying amounts of the drug's active ingredient. Before taking any particular brand, be sure to check the dosage your doctor prescribed with the amount per tablet. A standard aspirin tablet contains five grains or about 325 milligrams of the drug. Aspirin advertised as "arthritis strength" contains more aspirin per tablet than regular brands. In effect, if you take one "arthritis strength" aspirin, it's the same as taking more tablets of another brand that has a smaller amount of active ingredient in each pill.

Most common pain and cold remedies contain some amount of aspirin. You should not take one of these remedies on top of your regular aspirin dosage without consulting your doctor—you might overmedicate yourself without realizing it. Always read the labels of non-prescription drugs to see if they contain aspirin or other *salicylates.* Aspirin can be taken safely with some other medications—but not all other medications. Your doctor will tell you which drugs to avoid while you're taking aspirin.

Aspirin is available in different forms. Some have been developed for convenience, others are designed to reduce stomach distress—a common side effect of aspirin. There are liquid forms, buffered tablets, tablets with special coatings, and capsules that release aspirin very slowly into the bloodstream. Again, your doctor should tell you which form will best suit your needs.

Generic brands of aspirin usually cost less and work just as well as the more publicized brands.

xpensive way to buy aspirin is in bot- thousand tablets. If you find you tol- brand better than another, stay with that kind.

What About Aspirin Substitutes?

Tylenol, Datril, and other aspirin substitutes are *acetaminophens,* and they are used for the relief of headaches, fever, and mild pain. However, they do not contain the ingredients necessary to reduce the inflammation that most often comes with arthritis. You can substitute an *acetaminophen* for aspirin to help control pain, but not to reduce inflammation. Once again, your doctor can tell you if aspirin substitutes would be useful in your treatment.

Aspirin is frequently combined with an *acetaminophen* to relieve painful conditions other than arthritis. Sometimes, drugs such as caffeine, antihistamine, nasal drying agents, and sedatives are also added. These preparations are formulated specifically to treat colds or headaches, so they are not the best preparations for arthritis relief. If a combination of drugs is required, your doctor should prescribe each drug separately, and the dose of each should be targeted to your condition so that you receive the maximum benefit with a minimum of side effects.

What About Aspirin Liniments?

There are liquids and ointments that contain some form of aspirin. These are meant to be rubbed onto your skin over a painful area, such as a joint, for temporary pain relief.

One particular ointment called TEA has recently been promoted as an effective treatment for controlling the symptoms of arthritis.

According to Dr. Emmanuel Golden in a study he conducted, TEA was found to be at least as effective as aspirin while tending to provide pain relief more quickly. Also, it seemed to have fewer side effects and was therefore less likely to cause patients to abandon their program of treatment.

However, studies on the joint penetration of the aspirin in such preparations show that very little of the aspirin actually reaches the area of inflammation. Thus, the creams should only be used in addition to—not as a substitute for—the aspirin or other NSAIDs taken by mouth.

Your doctor should help you decide whether an ointment or rub would be beneficial for you and, if so, what kind to use.

What Are the Side Effects of Aspirin?

The most common side effect of aspirin is stomach irritation, which can include heartburn, indigestion, pain, nausea, and vomiting. Stomach irritation can lead to bleeding in the stomach which may cause its victim to have black stools. Taking aspirin with meals, with an antacid, or with a glass of milk can help avoid these symptoms. Coated aspirin tablets are also easier on the stomach.

It may help to avoid taking aspirin with alcohol or coffee, or with any other drinks that contain caffeine. Alcohol and caffeine make your stomach more susceptible to irritation. If you do experience stomach irritation when you take aspirin, tell your doctor. He may be able to recommend a less irritating preparation.

A few people develop asthma as a side effect to aspirin. Others may develop hay fever, nasal congestion, or hives. These people should never take aspirin or any other NSAID, nor should people with stomach or duodenal ulcers. If you suffer from any of these, ask your doctor to prescribe an effective aspirin substitute.

Aspirin can interfere with the blood's ability to clot. As a result, some people find they bruise easily when taking aspirin. People with significant bruising problems should be careful about taking aspirin.

High doses of aspirin and aspirin-like drugs may cause ringing in the ears and a slight deafness. If these side effects occur, call your doctor for instructions. If you can't reach him, cut your aspirin dosage by one tablet a day.

The following is a list of symptoms compiled by the Arthritis Foundation. If you notice that you have any of them, you may be experiencing a side effect from your medication. Consult your doctor.

- Rapid or deep breathing
- Ringing in the ears
- Decrease in hearing
- Drowsiness
- Nausea
- Vomiting
- Irritability

A note on aspirin advertising: Many ads for aspirin, especially those seen on television, make arthritis seem like a simple matter characterized by aches and pains. This is extremely misleading. Arthritis can be serious, the pain acute, and, if left untreated, the disease can lead to crippling and deformity.

Don't let advertising slogans lead you to believe that popping a few aspirins is a cure for your condition. There is much more to controlling arthritis than getting "immediate and wonderful relief" provided by a particular brand of aspirin. Only a physician can accurately and safely determine what kind of disease you may suffer from and prescribe the appropriate treatment.

Other Anti-Inflammatory Drugs

For the many people who cannot tolerate aspirin in continual large doses, it may not be the number one drug choice for treating their arthritis.

"The traditional view," says Dr. Jacques Caldwell, "is that aspirin should be the treatment of choice for any type of arthritis. But I practice in Florida where many of my arthritis patients are elderly. Many of them cannot tolerate aspirin in big enough doses."

Dr. Caldwell, clinical associate professor of medicine at the University of Florida, said that the average adult needs to take between twelve to eighteen five-grain aspirin tablets a day for the drug to be effective in the treatment of [rheumatoid] arthritis—especially the reduction of swelling.

If arthritis sufferers take less aspirin, then they don't receive the full benefit, says Dr. Caldwell.

In these cases, instead of aspirin, he suggests patients take *anti-inflammatory drugs* such as Naprosyn, Motrin, Clinoril, Nalfon, Tolectin, and other drugs described on the following pages.

Meclomen (meclofenamate): This drug has been found effective in reducing pain, the number of tender joints, and the degree of tenderness in each joint. Its most common side effects are diarrhea and abdominal pain.

Motrin and ***Rufen*** (ibuprofen): These drugs are used to treat both *rheumatoid arthritis* and *osteoarthritis.* They are prescribed in tablets and often given with other arthritis medications. Like aspirin, they fight the inflammation but can also cause stomach irritation.

Nalfon (fenoprofen): For *osteo-* and *rheumatoid arthritis* patients, this drug has been found effective in reducing joint pain, swelling, and duration of stiffness, as well as the spread of the disease. Its most common side effect is stomach irritation.

Naprosyn (naproxen): This drug comes in tablet form and is used to fight *osteo-* and *rheumatoid arthritis.* It helps control inflammation and disease activity. Its most common side effect is stomach irritation.

Clinoril (sulindac): This drug is an effective treatment for many forms of arthritis, including *rheumatoid arthritis, osteoarthritis, ankylosing spondylitis,* acute *gouty arthritis,* and acute painful shoulder due to *bursitis* or *tendinitis.* It can help control the symptoms of inflammation although it may cause stomach irritation in some patients.

Indocin (indomethacin): This drug is effective in treating *rheumatoid arthritis, gout,* certain forms of *osteoarthritis,* and *ankylosing spondylitis.* It is prescribed in oral capsules, and has widely differing effects on different disease symptoms. Therefore, it must be prescribed with special attention to the effects of your disease. The most common side effects are stomach irritation, headache, and dizziness.

Tolectin (tolmetin): Doctors prescribe this drug in tablet form and report that it is effective in treating *osteo-* and *rheumatoid arthritis* because it reduces the symptoms of inflammation. Its most common side effect is stomach irritation.

Butazoladin and ***Azolid*** (phenylbutazone): This drug is used for many painful joint conditions such as *ankylosing spondylitis, gout, tendinitis, bursitis,* and *fibrositis.* It should be used only in severe cases and under close medical supervision. Because it can have a serious effect on the blood cells, frequent laboratory tests are needed to monitor the drug's effects on your body. The drug is usually not used over a long period of time except in low dosages for people with *ankylosing spondylitis.* It is prescribed in tablet form, and its most common side effects are stomach irritation and retention of body fluid.

Feldene (piroxicam): The major advantage that this drug has over aspirin is that you need to take it only once a day. It is similar to the other anti-inflammatory drugs, but studies show that the fewer pills a person has to take, the more likely he is to take them. Its main side effect is stomach irritation.

Dolobid (diflunisal): This drug is chemically related to aspirin and has been found effective in fighting the pain caused by *osteoarthritis* as well as some nonarthritic symptoms. It has fewer side effects than aspirin, and its painkilling effects last twice as long. Dr. Caldwell, of the University of Florida, adds, "It's equivalent to a combination of aspirin and codeine or Tylenol and codeine. That's pretty significant pain relief!"

Steroid Drugs

One of the ironies of modern medicine is that some of the most effective treatments are the most dangerous. In every instance of serious illness—not just arthritis—doctors must weigh the merits of therapy against the possible dangers. Where modern drugs are concerned, a careful balance between helping and hurting must be struck. The patient and the doctor must discuss all the options: Are the risks worth taking? Is this the last possible course of action to alleviate the painful symptoms? What are the short-term risks versus the long term? Can the consequences of this therapy be worse than the problem it is supposed to solve?

The use of *steroid drugs* brings all these questions to the forefront. Steroids are powerful and potentially dangerous drugs. They are normally prescribed for people with arthritis *only when the disease does not respond to other drugs or therapies.* Steroids, which are hormones, are used to treat *lupus, rheumatoid arthritis, juvenile arthritis,* and other forms of arthritis.

The most commonly prescribed steroid is ***Prednisone.*** If your doctor prescribes steroids, do not stop taking the drug until he tells you to do so—the dose must be decreased very gradually to avoid complications. Although steroids are usually prescribed in tablet form, doctors will sometimes inject them directly into an affected joint for immediate, temporary relief. Steroids are often prescribed in conjunction with other drugs.

One particular but nonthreatening side effect sometimes seen in long-term steroid users is a swollen or a fat-looking "moon face." On rare occasions disturbances ranging from insomnia to depression can also result from steroid use. Steroids can also cause skin disorders, abnormal hair growth, a weakening of the bones, especially the spine (sometimes to the point where fractures occur for no apparent reason), stomach or intestinal ulcers, high blood pressure, cataracts, and even diabetes.

Aside from side effects, one of the primary dangers of using steroids in excessive amounts is that the drugs can mask symptoms of other illnesses. A patient receiving steroids may develop a serious infection and not know it. As a result, the unrecognized infection can progress to a point where it becomes very difficult to treat.

For all these reasons, many doctors are reluctant to prescribe steroids. Yet taken properly, for limited periods of time, they can be extremely valuable in controlling particularly painful arthritis flare-ups.

Some Other Drugs Used in Treating Arthritis

Chrysotherapy (Gold Therapy): Gold is an effective and medically approved treatment for *rheumatoid arthritis, juvenile arthritis* and *psoriatic arthritis.* In this treatment, people are usually given an injection of gold every week at first, and then the dosage is reduced to a shot twice a month. Since gold can be toxic, patients are watched closely. The body's response to gold therapy is very slow.

It may take twelve to fourteen weeks before you feel relief after the first injection. Gold, in the form of ***Solganol*** or ***Myochrysine,*** is given along with other medication. The most common side effect is a skin rash, and frequent laboratory tests must be performed to monitor the effect the gold has on your body because it can also damage the kidneys and the blood cells.

Cuprimine and ***Depen*** (Penicillamine): This drug is used to treat severe *rheumatoid arthritis.* It comes in either tablets or capsules and is prescribed by your doctor under the brand names Cuprimine or Depen. It also requires frequent monitoring. It can cause a wide variety of side effects and if you notice any, notify your doctor immediately. This drug may take as long as six months or more to produce any therapeutic or beneficial effects.

Plaquenil (Hydroxychloroquine): This antimalarial drug is used to treat the symptoms of *rheumatoid arthritis* and *systemic lupus.* It can reduce swelling, provide increased mobility, and can decrease the extent and severity of the rash that is associated with *lupus.*

Your body may take several weeks to respond to Plaquenil, and several months before the maximum benefit is felt. The most common side effects are a skin rash and damage to the retina of the eye. Regular eye examinations by an ophthalmologist are necessary for anyone taking this drug.

Drugs NOT Approved by the Food and Drug Administration (FDA)

Many arthritis patients are curious about drugs they've heard about that have not been approved by the FDA. The process by which the FDA approves a drug includes tests to determine its safety and effectiveness. Every drug is tested on animals first and then used in clinical tests in a hospital or laboratory on humans. In these clinical tests, subjects are under careful medical supervision so that any negative effects the drug might have will be observed and corrected immediately.

Taking drugs not yet approved by the FDA can be dangerous. It's like driving a car that hasn't been inspected; there are so many unknown and possibly dangerous conditions that can cause irreparable damage to your body. All the potential side effects of a drug must be examined before the drug is considered safe for humans and made available to the general public. There is good reason to wait for the approval of the FDA: An insufficiently tested drug could hurt you.

CHAPTER V

Arthritis Treatments: Exercise

AT FIRST IT MAY SOUND CRAZY, BUT EXERCISE IS A crucially important part of any comprehensive medical program for arthritis sufferers. Especially if you have never had arthritis, exercise seems like the least likely aspect of therapy. And if you have arthritis, it may seem humanly impossible. After all, how can someone with swollen and painful joints be expected to do exercise? Well, even those who are badly crippled can perform some kind of exercise—and maintain the function of their joints. And equally important, if you refuse to do any kind of exercising, you can only expect to get worse as time goes by.

When performed faithfully, exercise will limber up the joints, prevent additional debilitation from weakened muscles and deformities, and strengthen your ligaments, tendons and bones. Exercise programs can be developed to help anyone with arthritis. You should ask your doctor, physical therapist, or any other qualified professional to recommend a routine tailored to your specific needs and limitations. Do not try to create your own plan, because what is good for you when you are healthy and pain-free is not necessarily good for you when you have arthritis. If you borrow an exercise plan from someone else with the disease it is just as irresponsible as using someone else's medicine: It was prescribed specifically for him, not for you, and it can be very dangerous. The wrong exercises can make your arthritis worse and increase joint damage.

Why Do I Have to Exercise?

The simple truth is your body has to move. That's the reason why exercise is so important, for instance, after prolonged bed rest. Without motion and exercise, your muscles begin to atrophy, and your body grows weaker and weaker. According to the *Arthritis Exercise Book* by Semyon Krewer, many of the movements our bodies perform almost involuntarily are responses to a lack of movement. Examples of this include stretching, yawning, and turning over in bed.

Exercise and motion are particularly important for joints affected by arthritis. If you try not to use a particular joint because it is sore—it's only natural to protect an area that hurts—it will become even stiffer and more difficult to move. Eventually, the joint may become permanently rigid.

Exercise brings other, more general, benefits to the arthritis patient. The feeling of satisfaction and sense of achievement after exercise are open to everyone. They are signs of both physical and emotional well-being. Physically, the body has been loosened up, stretched, and moved into high gear. Emotionally, exercise has helped reduce mental stress and anxiety and improved the body's ability to relax.

In their book, the *Arthritis Helpbook: What You Can Do for Your Arthritis,* Drs. Kate Lorig and James F. Fries explain that more specific benefits of exercise for those with arthritis include "increased strength and flexibility of the muscles and ligaments that surround a joint. Research has shown that exercise helps to maintain or even increase the strength of bone."

Exercise can also help transport vital nutrients through your body. Tissues have blood vessels which bring nutrients to them, but movement is necessary to carry the proper nutrients through joint fluids into joint cartilage, and to carry waste products out of the cartilage.

One point cannot be emphasized too strongly: If you do not exercise a joint, you will lose strength, mobility, and function in that joint. If you have already suffered a loss of function in a joint, you didn't lose that movement in a day, so you can't realistically expect to regain it in one exercise session. You must expect slow progress, especially if you have severe arthritis or your joints have been gradually stiffening over a long period of time. Don't be discouraged if your progress seems slow—stick to your exercise program and you will see positive results.

Don't exercise to the point of increased pain. If a particular movement seems to make the pain more severe, eliminate it from your routine until you can discuss it with your doctor or physical therapist. You need to learn to use pain as a guide throughout your experience with arthritis—it can send you important signals. Just be sure you are not hiding behind it to avoid following your treatment.

When Should I Exercise?

Experts agree that ordinarily you should try to exercise twice a day for about fifteen minutes each time. Sporadic or occasional exercise can result in painful, strained muscles and ligaments. An inflamed joint, one that is red, hot, and tender to the touch, should not be strenuously exercised, but it can be gently moved through its range of motion every day.

Choose the best times of day and the best places for you to exercise. Make these exercise periods part of your daily routine. The times when you usually have the least pain and stiffness, don't feel tired, and your medicine is having the most effect, are the best times to set aside for your exercise program. And remember to start slowly when you begin to exercise.

The Different Kinds of Exercise

Exercises for the person who has arthritis are generally more gentle than conventional vigorous exercise. Some, called *active exercises,* are performed without any outside assistance and often under the supervision of a doctor or physical therapist. Others, called *passive exercises,* require that a therapist move the patient's hand, arm, leg, or other afflicted area.

Assistive exercises fall somewhere in between because they are performed with the help of an assistant. Exercises of this kind are used to increase a joint's range of movement and to build up muscle strength. For example, a patient who cannot completely straighten his knees may eventually regain that ability after a therapist has repeatedly helped to move the knees and legs into a fully extended position.

Gentle daily range of motion exercise for all affected joints is required to keep joints limber. For instance, stretching your fingers on the flat surface of a tabletop will help prevent your fingers from becoming stiff or fixed in one position. These exercises, which you can easily do while talking on the phone or working at your desk, should be performed several times a day.

Doing the ROM Hop

Imagine! A dance for arthritis! It was developed to help encourage people with arthritis to do their exercises. ROM refers to *range-of-motion,* and it is a series of flowing and graceful movements to be done while sitting or standing up. It has been praised as an exciting way to get arthritic joints moving and keep them moving.

ROM takes one of the most gentle Oriental martial arts called T'ai Chi, and combines it with standard arthritis exercises performed to the words of a poem. The leader of the dance uses the words of the poem to lead a group through the slow and flowing exercises. You can also get a cassette so that you can do the movements alone at home.

The poem can employ any subject as long as it is relaxing and not too energetic. The dancers, for instance, may see themselves on a warm and sunny beach, bathing in soothing water. As the poem takes us to the water's edge, it may say, "Stepping deeper into the water I feel the sun warm my head and neck . . ." and the dancers roll their heads around in a circular motion. ROM emphasizes breathing and balance, as well as typical arthritis exercises.

According to Dr. Diane Harlow, one of the creators of the dance, and director of occupational therapy and speech services at St. Mary's Hospital Medical Center in Madison, Wisconsin, the big advantage of the ROM dance over the other exercising routines is that it requires only seven minutes to perform—and it's fun.

If you are interested in this form of exercise you can consult your local chapter of the Arthritis Foundation to see if it offers classes in the ROM dance.

Striking a Balance

As we mentioned before, your exercise plan must be designed for you, otherwise you can cause further damage to the areas already affected by arthritis. For instance, *osteoarthritis* can cause what are called *flexion contractures*—a stiffening of joints into a locked position. A person with *flexion contracture* of the hip, for example, cannot stand up straight or lie flat in bed. In such a situation, exercises might be prescribed which emphasize efforts to achieve full motion of the involved hip.

Dr. McDuffie, Medical Director of the Arthritis Foundation, points out, "If you do too much exercise, the joints will flare up and become worse. If you do too little exercise, the joints will become contracted and deformed. You have to strike a proper balance."

Children with arthritis should be encouraged to be active. They should be allowed to join in other children's games as much as their physical conditions will allow. If you are in doubt about just how much physical activity is right for your child's condition, talk to your doctor.

For some children, ordinary play activity may be the only exercise required. For the majority, however, specifically planned exercises of their own are necessary. Your doctor, or someone he recommends, can teach your child and you how to move joints through their range of motion.

Parents of school-age arthritis victims should meet with the child's teachers. Discuss your child's need to get up and walk around the classroom every so often to prevent his joints from becoming stiff while sitting at his desk. You might suggest to the teacher that your child run errands or distribute classroom papers—that's a good way to keep the stiffness from settling in.

In some cases, if motion has been lost in a joint, if the joint has become fixed in one bent position, or if muscles have become weak, your child may need special exercises. A physical therapy program should be worked out by you, your doctor or physical therapist, and your child.

As with adults, excessive motion or activity can cause inflammation to flare. Children can usually tell if they've done too much by the way they feel the next day, but you must learn to observe your child's reactions carefully. Children may not always tell you how they really feel and many children seem to be less sensitive to pain than adults. Sometimes they push themselves too hard trying to keep up with their playmates. On the other hand, children sometimes learn to use fatigue and soreness as a way to avoid doing things they don't want to do. Again, as with adults, a proper balance must be reached and maintained.

A General Exercise Plan

The following plan has been put together by The ENQUIRER based on information provided by Tufts-New England Medical Center, the Arthritis Foundation, the National Institute of Arthritis, Metabolism, and Digestive Diseases and leading rheumatologists. It is an easy-to-follow exercise program of gentle, daily exercises you can do at home to prevent muscle deterioration, increase strength—even relieve depression by making you feel better about yourself physically.

Always remember that exercises should not be done without a doctor's or a therapist's approval, and do not exercise beyond the point of pain. Here are some simple movements you can do at home that can be helpful in relieving arthritic pain in specific joints.

Wrist and Hand

This is one of the areas most commonly affected by arthritic pain and stiffness. You can usually relieve your symptoms with these exercises:

1. *Immerse your hand in a bowl of warm water* and:
   - Slowly and gently open and close your fingers several times.
   - Bend fingers at knuckles several times.
   - Touch the finger tips with the thumb.

2. *Place the palms of your hand on a table,* spread your fingers and press down gently to stretch them.

3. *Place your palms on a table,* gently lift each finger, then all the fingers together.

Experts warn against squeezing a rubber ball or ball of wool as exercise unless your doctor specifically approves of this. Knitting, sewing, crocheting and other household tasks *are not* substitutes for exercises.

There is no home treatment for more serious hand and wrist disorders. If your fingers start to "lock" when the hand is closed in a fist or if a finger or thumb can only be straightened with difficulty, consult your doctor or therapist.

Ankle, Foot and Toes

This is another area commonly affected by arthritis. Anyone with painful arthritic feet can strengthen the ankle, foot, and toe muscles by doing these exercises ten times each:

1. *Lying flat, rotate the foot* clockwise and then counter-clockwise.

2. *Lying flat, bend the foot* forward and then backward. You will get even more relief if you do these first two exercises in the morning, sitting in the bathtub.

3. *While standing, try to grasp the carpet* with the toes and then relax them.

4. *Push the ball of the foot* against a fixed bar or bed rail while lying flat. Alternately bend and spread the toes.

In addition to the exercise, you can ease foot pain by wearing shoes that fit properly. Don't wear shoes with more than a one-inch heel.

Knee

Some knee pain is very common in arthritis, particularly among athletes and overweight people who spend a lot of time on their feet. Don't ignore it. See a doctor right away to have it diagnosed.

The quadriceps muscle along the front of the thigh can become thin and weak within a short time and can cause the knee to become bent. Bicycle-type exercises or other strenuous activity can worsen the condition.

Here are some preventive measures you can take to keep this muscle strong:

1. *Lose weight* if you're overweight.
2. *Lie flat on a bed,* keeping the affected leg straight. Tighten the muscle on top of the knee and try to push the back of the knee down against the bed. Hold for a count of five. Repeat ten times.
3. *Repeat the same exercise,* lifting the tightened leg up and keeping it as straight as possible, for a count of five. Then slowly lower the leg.
4. *Repeat the same exercise* using a one or two pound sandbag on the ankle if the leg can handle it. Increase to five pounds when you're able.

Elbow

Many forms of arthritis cause symptoms in the elbow. These simple exercises help maintain elbow function:

1. *Stand with the arm straight down,* palm forward, and grasp a roll of bandage or cloth in your hand. Bend the arm at the elbow up toward you while squeezing the roll. Relax your hand while straightening the arm. *Do not use this exercise if you have arthritis in the hand as well as the wrist.*
2. *Repeat the exercise,* this time with your palm facing behind you.

Do each exercise fifteen times, two or three times a day.

Neck

A painful stiff neck often responds well to home treatment.

1. *Try sleeping flat* on your back with one pillow beneath your neck.
2. *Examine your life* for emotional problems that may be linked to your pain. Stress and anxiety can worsen a stiff neck that is due to muscular spasm and not arthritis.
3. *Adjust the height* of your desk chair so you don't have to hold your head too far forward. If you

spend long hours at a desk, your pain caused by leaning over from a chair thầ high.

Shoulders

Many different diseases associated with arthritis can cause shoulder pain, which usually appears when you raise your arm forward or above your head while dressing.

Here are exercises you can do for fifteen minutes, two or three times daily:

1. *While standing, bend over at the waist* and dangle your arm straight down with the fingers straight. Now gently make small movements in a circle with your arm, gradually increasing the size of the circle.
2. *Stand up straight with your arms at your side.* Bend the elbow at a right angle and turn your arm out to the side and then back in front of you. Now try reaching across your body and touching the opposite shoulder.
3. *Lie on a bed with arms at your side.* While keeping your painful arm flat on the bed, move it to shoulder level and then over your head. When it loosens up and the pain decreases, try lifting the arm straight out in front of you toward the ceiling and then swinging it backward over your head.
4. *While standing, grasp a broomstick* horizontally from side to side with both hands spread apart

and raise it as high as you can. Still holding the broom, swing your arms from side to side.

5. *While lying or standing, grasp both hands* behind your neck and pull the elbows apart.

Hip

For arthritis symptoms in the hip, try these self-treatment steps in conjunction with your doctor's advice:

1. *Limit walking* and stair climbing.
2. *Use a rubber-tipped cane* on the side opposite the pain.
3. *Lose excess weight.*

Back

A backache that is minor in the morning but gets worse as the day wears on will often respond to home treatment. Try these measures:

1. *Sleep on a firm mattress.* A three-quarter-inch board between your mattress and the box spring will make it firmer.
2. *Don't sit or stand for too long.*
3. *Avoid jumping out of bed,* or rising suddenly from a chair.
4. *Keep your back straight* when lifting things, letting your knees and hips bear the weight.

Water Babies

One of the most popular forms of exercise for people with arthritis is swimming. Whether you actually swim laps or just perform exercises depends on your personal abilities.

Water is an ideal exercise environment. Its buoyancy lessens the effects of gravity—your body is weightless—on your joints, and the water itself provides a gentle resistance to your movements. These two characteristics allow you to exercise your joints more completely without pain, so you are more likely to see results sooner. And most people who have arthritis report that since exercising in a swimming pool is far more enjoyable, they're more likely to stick to their exercise routine.

In addition, exercising in a pool can have social benefits. If you go with a group of people who also have arthritis you can enjoy the camaraderie of exercising together. Or you can go to a pool alone to get a change of scenery and perspective.

With all these positive aspects in mind, the Arthritis Foundation and the YMCA have joined forces to develop an exciting new arthritis exercise program. It is called the Arthritis Aquatics Program (AAP), and it is practiced in a pool in shoulder-deep warm water; you don't have to know how to swim to be able to reap its benefits. The exercises are only done under the supervision of a trained AAP leader. As a result you must contact your local chapter of the Arthritis Foundation for information about this program.

Here is a brief look at the program and why it was developed. According to the Foundation's Medical

Director, Dr. McDuffie, "The program provides people with an easy way to help beat the pain of arthritis. The buoyancy and warmth of the water—which is heated to between 83 and 88 degrees—relieves pain and stiffness, making exercise easier. And exercise is vital for the person with arthritis."

The program contains sixty-five exercises and activities—but they are geared to each individual's own pace and specific needs. Participants work out two or three times a week for thirty to forty-five minutes each time, over a six- to ten-week period. They are under the supervision of an instructor-lifeguard. The AAP includes dozens of exercises to improve your range of motion. They focus on trunk stretching, toe and ankle rotation, wrist and finger presses, knee bends, breathing, and a large variety of other areas.

The exercises are simple—and they get rave reviews from the people with arthritis who use them. "When I get out of the water, I feel like I can do anything," says eighty-one-year-old Marion Schryver of Whittier, California, who works out three times a week. "The warm water relieves my pain and stiffness. And the program makes me feel so much better. I love it!"

The Arthritis Aquatics Program is available at about one hundred places nationwide. Contact your local Arthritis Foundation chapter to find out whether it is available near you. In addition, nearly half of the YMCAs around the country offer similar warm water exercise programs. Check with your local Y to see if one is available.

If no program is available in your area, ask your doctor or therapist to design one for you. Remember to check with your doctor or therapist before starting any new exercise program.

CHAPTER VI

Arthritis Treatments: Surgery

PERHAPS THE GREATEST RECENT PROGRESS IN THE treatment of arthritis has been made in the field of surgery. It is now possible to replace a large number of arthritic joints (not just the hip) with artificial joints made of plastic and metal, and held in place with cement. Hip replacements are now successful about 90 percent of the time, and last up to ten years or even more. This kind of operation comes under the field of *orthopedic* surgery, and is called *arthroplasty*.

Surgery always involves a certain risk, and only you and your physician can decide whether you should take this risk. In some cases, drugs and exercise do not relieve your pain or improve your mobility enough to allow you to have the quality of life you feel you must have to be happy, or to perform the job you work at. Under these and other circumstances surgery is an option—and a very effective one.

Replacement of the hip joint is nearly routine surgery today. Knee replacement was considered experimental a decade ago and now is almost commonplace. Finger joints, shoulders, and elbows are all becoming areas where surgery can be used successfully. But you should know that even the most successful surgery cannot improve your condition to the point where you can play football again or run in marathons. The goal of surgery is to relieve pain and improve the usefulness of a joint. It is not a miracle cure.

Reasons for Surgery

As we have said before, inflammation and the deterioration of bone and cartilage can cause joints, tendons, and their coverings to be damaged or pulled out of place, resulting in pain, impaired function, and physical deformity. Any one of these problems may lead you to consider surgery.

Pain is a constant companion to anyone who has severe arthritis. It can often be relieved by rest, heat and cold therapy, exercise, and medication. But if this combination of treatments fails to provide adequate relief, you may want to consider surgery.

When a joint such as a hip, knee, or ankle becomes totally nonfunctional as a result of arthritis, your ability to carry out your daily activities may be seriously impaired. If this happens, your doctor may recommend surgery to replace or reconstruct the damaged joint.

Although surgery can usually relieve pain, the restoration of joint movement and function is less predictable. Cosmetic improvement in deformed joints depends largely upon the joints involved—for example, surgery nearly always improves the appearance of arthritic hands. Your doctor will carefully evaluate how much pain relief, restored joint function, and improvement in appearance you can reasonably expect before suggesting surgery.

Arguments Against Surgery

The decision to have surgery is a difficult one. Your doctor, after consulting with a surgeon, may tell you that surgery is not likely to provide the benefits you seek. Even if your doctor tells you that surgery may help you, you should be aware of the drawbacks and potential complications.

In any operation, there is always the danger of infection. Any bacterial infection you may currently have, such as bronchitis or a bladder infection, must be cleared up before surgery is performed. If it isn't eliminated, the infection may spread to the healing joint and cause serious problems.

Other conditions that must be evaluated include the possibility of triggering serious heart disease or breathing problems. Surgery is a strain even on the healthiest of people. Since arthritis surgery is elective—planned ahead of time rather than done on an emergency basis—it is important that your general health be excellent.

Overweight people may be particularly poor risks for surgery, because any excess weight puts additional stress on the heart and lungs. The operation is also technically more difficult for the surgeon if there is a lot of excess fatty tissue to cut through. And, in the case of surgery on a weight-bearing joint such as a hip or knee, recovery of the joint is hindered by the stress of extra weight. Excess body weight also makes it harder to perform the exercises that are essential for strengthening a joint after surgery.

You must be realistic about what to expect from surgery. Although your doctor has no way to predict the exact results of surgery, you should limit your expectations. For example, when a joint is severely deformed, surgery will usually improve its range of motion and provide some relief from pain. But you will not have as perfect a joint as you had before arthritis.

Realize also that you will have to follow a strict course of treatment *after* surgery. Unlike surgery to remove a diseased organ such as an appendix, the success of arthritis surgery may not be immediately apparent. The operation itself is only the first step toward restoration of a joint. After the operation, the amount of effort you put into the recovery process can mean the difference between success and failure. If you've had trouble following your doctor's advice about medication, diet, and exercise, you may not be a good candidate for surgery. The recovery period is critical to the surgery's success. If you don't think you are fully committed to carrying out a prescribed course of post-surgical rest, exercise, medication, and diet, it might not be worth going through all the pain and expense of surgery.

Questions to Ask Your Doctor About Surgery

1. What treatments can I try as alternatives to surgery?
2. Can you briefly and simply explain the surgical procedure?
3. How long will the surgery take?
4. What risks are involved in the procedure?
5. Will I need a blood transfusion?
6. What kind of anesthesia will I be given to put me to sleep during the operation?
7. How much improvement can I expect from the surgical procedure?
8. Will any additional surgery be needed?
9. What other doctors will be involved during surgery and the recovery period?
10. How often has the surgeon performed this procedure?
11. May I speak with another patient who has undergone this particular operation?
12. How long should I expect to stay in the hospital?
13. How long do I have to stay in bed after surgery?
14. How long before physical therapy is started?
15. Is physical therapy covered by insurance?
16. Will I need any special equipment for physical therapy?
17. Will I need to arrange for special help at home after surgery?
18. What kind of pain and how much pain should I expect after the operation?
19. What medications will I be taking at home, and for how long?

20. What restrictions will there be on my activities, and for how long?
21. How often will I need follow-up appointments?

There are many other questions you will probably want to ask. Be sure that you do.

Five Kinds of Arthritis Surgery

The following comments briefly describe different kinds of arthritis surgery. They provide some background information which may help you with discussing surgery with your doctor. Some surgical techniques are being phased out as popular solutions because as research continues, more reliable procedures with long-term results are being discovered.

Synovectomy is the removal of the diseased *synovium* (the lining of a joint) to reduce pain and swelling experienced by people with *rheumatoid arthritis.* Unfortunately, the *synovium* usually grows back after surgery, bringing the symptoms back with it. This operation is most often performed on the knee, the wrist, and the hand joints. It can also be effective on the shoulder, elbow, foot, and ankle. If the operation is performed early in the course of the disease, before bone and cartilage have been eroded, it may extend the functional life of the joint in addition to relieving pain.

Osteotomy is the correction of a deformity by cutting and then resetting a bone in the proper alignment. This procedure allows the bone to heal into a normal position.

Resection is the removal of a bone, or of part of a bone. A resection may be performed when the damaged joints in the feet make walking difficult. Painful bunions are also removed by resection.

Arthrodesis or *Bone Fusion* has been used to relieve pain, usually in the ankles and wrist. The procedure involves fusing or joining two small bones together. It is a severe remedy and is recommended only when joints stop working altogether. Fusion results in a rigid "locking" of the joint in place.

Arthroplasty is the rebuilding of joints by resurfacing or relining the ends of bones where cartilage has worn away and has caused destruction to the bones. Arthroplasty also refers to the replacement of an entire joint with a prosthesis, an artificial replacement for a body part.

The Hips

Several forms of arthritis of the hips can cause constant pain and difficulty in sitting and walking. Dramatic improvements have taken place in correcting these problems. Hip replacement techniques have brought relief from pain and have restored joint function to thousands of people, including actress Katharine Hepburn.

Both the condition of the bones and the age of the patient are considered before a doctor decides which surgical technique will be most successful.

According to the National Institutes of Health, more

than 100,000 hip replacements are performed in the United States each year. The worldwide figure may be as high as 300,000. Of the 100,000 Americans who undergo hip replacement surgery each year, 90 percent report improved range of motion, 95 percent report that they can walk greater distances than they could before surgery, and 82 percent report relief of pain.

Though total hip replacement is perhaps the most dramatic and effective advance in surgery as far as arthritis patients are concerned, the procedure is not perfect, nor can every patient benefit from the operation. Eventually the bond between the artificial joint and the bone to which it is glued begins to break down, and slippage becomes increasingly frequent after seven to ten years. When this happens, a new replacement must be inserted. Surgeons are attempting to design replacements that will hold without slipping, but not enough time has passed to determine whether the new porous-coated prosthesis will last longer. Another complication of hip replacement is infection. Though infection is happening less and less, when it occurs the prosthesis must be removed.

An artificial hip made of metal and plastic can't restore anyone's life to normal. Although the artificial hip can make pain-free motion possible, a patient cannot expect to return to the way of life that he knew before the onset of arthritis. Here are some guidelines that can help you determine whether you might be a good candidate for hip replacement. Are you:

- a person of any age with severe *rheumatoid arthritis* of the hip?
- a person fifty years of age or older with severe *osteoarthritis* in one or both hips?

- a person with an abnormally developed hip?
- a person with severe traumatic arthritis—arthritis caused by an injury to the hip?

If any of these descriptions apply to you, ask your doctor about surgery.

The Hand and Wrist

Arthritic deformities of the wrists and hands can cause impaired functioning as well as pain. If conventional treatment fails to improve the functioning of deformed hands, if simple tasks such as holding a fork or fastening a button cause pain, surgery may be a solution. In addition, some arthritis victims are very sensitive about the appearance of their deformed hands, so the cosmetic effect of corrective surgery can also improve their overall sense of well-being.

Sometimes surgery is performed to tighten or relax the tension exerted by the pull of tendons in hands, a procedure that can improve manual dexterity.

When the wrist is painful, there are several procedures that may offer relief. *Fusion,* also called *arthrodesis,* eliminates the wrist's range-of-motion, but often relieves pain and increases the hand's stability. Sometimes *resection* of one of the bones in the wrist may reduce pain and improve motion.

The Shoulder

If exercise and medication don't adequately control pain in the shoulder, your doctor may suggest that you consider a *synovectomy.*

Total joint replacement often relieves pain, but usually restores only a limited range of motion to the shoulder. This is a difficult operation and recovery requires many months.

The Ankle and Foot

Since the feet and ankles bear the body's full weight, impaired function and pain in the lower extremities can be severely disabling. If therapy and the use of braces and special shoes fail to relieve the problem, surgery may be considered.

One of the most common surgical procedures performed on arthritic ankles is the *fusion* of bones. Replacement of the ankle is not yet a satisfactory operation. *Resection,* or cutting off the ends of bones, is performed when the pain in the feet is severe enough to prevent the patient from walking. Toe deformities can be corrected by a number of surgical procedures including *resection, fusion,* and replacement of toe joints.

The Knee

The knee is an unstable, weight-bearing joint that is especially vulnerable to stress-related injuries. When conventional arthritis treatments fail to alleviate symptoms in the knee, your doctor may recommend a number of surgical procedures including *synovectomy* or total joint replacement.

No surgery can restore a knee to its pre-arthritic levels of flexibility and weight-bearing capacity. But the procedures do offer relief from the most pressing problems of pain, instability, and loss of mobility.

The Elbow

Elbow surgery is usually performed to relieve pain and stiffness which can severely limit the use of the hand. A *synovectomy,* with or without *resection,* can provide this relief only when the problem is not the result of *osteoarthritis* or injury. Resurfacing or joint replacement are other possible methods of restoring movement to the elbow.

After the Operation

Depending on the type of surgery you've had, your physician will prescribe a period of rest, physical therapy, and limited activity suited to your condition.

In addition to days or even weeks of rest, you may need to use splints, a cane, or crutches before you're able to perform your usual tasks. You will also have to follow a special exercise routine to regain the strength of the joints affected by surgery.

How Much Will It Cost?

A number of factors—the surgeon's fee, surgical procedure, daily hospital costs, physical therapy requirements, etc., determine the cost of corrective surgery. But, as you probably already know, no surgery or hospital stay is inexpensive. You will need to check with

The Bionic Grandmother

Rose Iacoma is a medical marvel—incredibly, every major joint in her body has been replaced with artificial ones! The sixty-eight-year-old grandmother, who has had severe arthritis for over a decade, has new shoulders, new elbows, new hips, new knees—and a new lease on life!

"I used to be in constant pain," revealed Rose, of Union, New Jersey, who had a mind-boggling fifteen operations in six years. "Before the operations, I could hardly walk. I couldn't comb my hair or brush my teeth or even wash my face. Now I can even walk without pain. And everyone calls me the Bionic Woman."

Dr. Charles Neer, of New York's Columbia Presbyterian Medical Center, performed some of the operations and said, "Rose is unique. I don't know of anyone else who has had all his major joints replaced."

Agonizing arthritis pain struck in Rose's hips in the early 1970s. Her doctor's treatment did not seem to work and so finally he suggested that she have her hip joints replaced or plan on being confined to a wheelchair in the future. At first, Rose was frightened but as the pain got worse she didn't know where else to turn for relief. In May 1976 her doctor replaced both hip joints and "For the first time in years, I could walk without pain," Rose remembered. "Then in 1978 I could hardly lift my shoulders without dagger-like pains shooting through them." That is when Dr. Neer replaced both her shoulder joints. Two years later, Rose's right elbow joint was replaced, followed by both knees and another elbow. "Now I'm pain free!" Rose proclaimed later. "I thank God every night for the freedom from pain."

your doctor, insurance company, and, if you qualify, with Medicaid or Medicare concerning the extent of your coverage. Check the costs and coverage before you schedule any surgery to avoid any unpleasant surprises when you receive your bill. If you've spent time in a hospital during the year, the year's benefits may be used up and your surgery will have to be postponed until your benefits are in full force again. The best rule of thumb, after you have checked out all of the known expenses, is to figure it will cost even more.

CHAPTER VII

Emotional Health and Arthritis

AN OVERALL SENSE OF WELL-BEING IS A CRITICAL ingredient in everyone's life. It can be defined as happiness, being at peace with oneself, satisfaction with life, or simply a general feeling of contentment and fulfillment. Basically, this is what we all strive for in our lives. When we look beyond financial security, owning our own house or car, raising a family, or working at a job we like, we look to happiness as the measure of our success in living. Typically, an illness is seen as a barrier, or end, to happiness. But this just is not so. If you have arthritis, the most important joys and pleasures of life are still there for the taking. The ways in which you go about enjoying them and finding them may be altered—even different—but the satisfactions, achievements, and fulfillment are much the same as they have always been.

The Emotional Impact

Learning that you have arthritis is a shock. Sure, you knew something was wrong because of your symptoms, but now it has a name. At first you may experience a feeling of relief that you haven't got a life-threatening illness. Then you may forget your initial relief and begin to think about just what it means to have arthritis and how it will affect your life in the short term and over a longer period of time. You may want to read up on facts about the particular form of arthritis you have. Certainly you will have questions for your doctor. But one of the first major hurdles you will face in the process of accepting your diagnosis is the uncertainty of just what to expect in the future.

First, let's establish what is certain about arthritis. Then we can tackle the uncertainties. Because arthritis is a chronic disease, it can last for a long period of time, depending upon what form of arthritis you have. Generally the symptoms can be controlled through a treatment program which includes medication and exercise. If you neglect any part of your whole treatment program you can expect further damage to your body to take place. Arthritis medications are given to relieve pain and inflammation. These medications have to be taken on a regular daily schedule in order to be effective, and this means you should take them even when your symptoms are vague or seem to be receding. In addition to medication and exercise, hot and cold therapy, rest and relaxation techniques, and joint protection will help you to manage pain.

Now let's look at the uncertainties. It is difficult to anticipate how you will feel day-to-day, week-to-week. You may worry that you won't feel up to making dinner or going to your child's school play. You may be angry or depressed because you feel you have lost control of your life. You may feel sadness that your life has changed and you can't turn back the clock. These feelings are entirely natural. A chronic disease brings with it all these emotions and more. It will take time to adjust. It will take time to learn to live with uncertainty. And it may take you awhile to learn to express all these feelings to others, whether they are family members or friends, counselors or doctors. Airing your feelings is terribly important. Getting them out in the open, examining them with the help of others, and putting to rest unwarranted fears and anxieties will help you not only emotionally, but physically as well.

How you feel about your life, yourself, your family, your body (and the changes it is going through) can affect how you deal with your illness. Your emotional health can affect your physical health. Your attitude toward your arthritis can influence your treatment and its effectiveness. Remember during this period that you aren't alone. There are people who can help you to adjust to living with arthritis. You may find a social worker or psychologist easier to talk to, or other people with arthritis may offer you the kind of support you need. Your doctor can offer advice on professional help. Your local chapter of the Arthritis Foundation will aid you in finding local clubs and support groups nearby.

The Impact on Your Family

Even as you continue the process of adjustment and acceptance within yourself, you need to begin to look beyond yourself. Arthritis has happened not only to *you,* it has also happened to *your family*. If you and your family have been faced with a serious problem in the past you have probably experienced a drawing together to meet the crisis. This coming together for support and strength is probably as old as civilization itself. And even if you haven't experienced it before, the intrusion of illness into a family can be an incredibly unifying force.

This doesn't mean, of course, that other family members don't share your fears or anxieties. They also share your need to understand your disease, to learn as much about it as you learn, and to learn to accept it even as you are discovering how to accept it yourself. Communication is a critical element in this process. You will need to tell your family when you need help and when you want to fend for yourself. You will need to involve your whole family in your treatment program, including explanations by your doctor or therapist about your need for exercise and rest. You can work together on adjusting the physical aspects of your house so that your home environment is easy for you to move around in and work in. Furniture can be moved, cabinets and counters can be altered. And you can share many chores as a family which you used to do on your own, like making dinner, cleaning up the dishes, washing the car, ironing, doing the laundry, and making beds. These "community" activities can bring a special closeness to your family. Each member can find his own special usefulness in your rearranged household, along with the comfort of simply helping each other.

At first, your children may find it hard to adjust to having a parent with arthritis. Clearly each child will react differently depending upon age and personality. Encourage your children to talk with you and tell you how they feel about your illness. And be sure to talk with them about how you feel emotionally and physically. If you are in pain, or your joints feel stiff and inflamed, and you ask them to do some extra chores to help you out, they should know the reason. After all, their lives are changing, too. They are expected to take on added responsibilities and they need to know why.

The Impact on Your Job

If you catch a cold or get the flu it can affect how you do your job. You might stay at home for a day or two to recuperate. Or you might go on working but at a slower pace to compensate for how you feel. Usually you wouldn't be worried about being sick for a couple of days because your coworkers and your boss would all understand; everybody gets sick once in a while. But when you have a chronic illness there may be many subtle changes involving your job. It is very important for you to get used to your arthritis before you can evaluate whether, or how, it will affect your job. At first, if you experience a flare-up of symptoms you may feel panicky about how you are going to do your work.

The first rule is *wait.* Don't jump to any conclusions. Don't make any decisions until you are feeling better.

When you and your doctor have established a treatment program, and you have learned what you can and cannot do in a practical sense, and you feel that you have started to gain a perspective on how to live with your particular set of symptoms, then talk with your employer about your arthritis. Help him or her to understand your condition. A lot will depend on how you communicate with your boss, the kind of job you have, and how you feel about your job. Often, some simple adjustments will be all that's needed for you to continue working. Things like a rest break, a new chair, a rearranged work area, and helpful tools for opening file cabinets and drawers, typing, writing and the like are often all it takes in the way of modifications. An occupational therapist can help you and your boss with the changes.

It is also possible that the nature of your job may need to be altered. You will have to talk with your employer about the possibilities of changing your responsibilities or the number of days you work and whether some flexibility can be put into your schedule. It can be helpful to contact the Department of Vocational Rehabilitation in your state for advice on how to adjust your job to your needs and abilities. Clearly, a lot will depend upon your employer's attitude, as well as your own.

In some cases your job may simply be too physically demanding for you to continue doing. This may be the time to try something new. Maybe you have always wanted to get into a new line of work but were afraid to try it. Now is the time you can seek retraining without feeling guilty or foolhardy about it. Again, go to a Department of Vocational Rehabilitation counselor in your state for advice. It may even be that you don't need new training. A counselor can tell you how to adapt the skills you already have to a new job, and even how to go about getting financing for retraining.

Remember to give yourself some time. Discuss all your options with the people around you, including your family and employer. Weigh the pros and cons carefully for each step you take. Plan ahead and establish interim goals as you make changes in your life. As you reach a goal, sit down and evaluate where you are now, and whether your plans need to be altered. Don't just look to the future either, look at your accomplishments and enjoy your successes—you have earned them.

The Impact on Physical Activity

Whether you love to cook or knit, or find running and a friendly game of tennis the high points of your "free time," arthritis will affect your ability to do some of the things you have enjoyed in the past. It would be the same if you had sustained an injury to your wrist or had torn the ligaments in your knee. Even the natural process of aging places restrictions on what you can do. We all face this inevitable decline in our strength, agility, and performance. If you have arthritis, don't let your feelings of frustration and anger—even guilt—trap you into a corner of isolation and loneliness.

There will be many, many things you can still do if you will only use some planning and ingenuity. If your hands and wrists are affected by arthritis, and lifting heavy pots and pans is too painful, you have two choices: You can quit doing something you love, or you can figure out a way around your limitations. Lightweight aluminum cookware is widely available. Plastic and stainless-steel mixing bowls weigh very little. Electric mixers can do the stirring and kneading you find too painful. And when the cake must finally be put into the oven, ask for some help. No one's going to mind spending a minute lifting the cake tins in or out of the oven.

There is no doubt that sporting activities, which place stress and strain on your joints, are going to be difficult to do. And they can hurt you physically. If you want to continue playing tennis or running, you must first consult your doctor. You can also switch to another sport, such as swimming, which gives you the exercise you need without the stress to your joints. Don't forget coaching either. Ball players, tennis and soccer players, golfers, and basketball stars all reach a time when they have to move on to another career. Often they choose coaching because it keeps them near the sport they love and allows them to teach what they have spent their lives learning. Coaching your son's soccer team, being first-base coach for the local softball team, or forming a nearby tennis club are all ways to involve yourself in pursuits you have long loved, but can no longer do yourself.

The possibilities are nearly endless if you just put your mind to it and learn to plan ahead. Fatigue is often a factor present in anyone with arthritis. You may feel unusually tired. Or you may tire easily when you perform routine tasks. Or the pain you experience in connection with your condition may tire you out. This is normal when you have arthritis, although it does vary in intensity from person to person. If the demands of your job were exhausting you, you would try to get more rest, get to bed earlier, plan fewer activities and chores on the weekend. If running your household became too hectic, and you found you were tired all the time, then you would try to decrease your workload by sharing the chores with other family members, taking a "vacation" for a week from all but the most critical daily duties, or finding some other way to rest up. Well, you should use this same process of planning, resting, and sharing when you have arthritis.

Any illness will make demands on your body which are greater and more tiring than when you were entirely well. Arthritis is an illness, and you must learn to accept the fact that you will often not have the energy and stamina you once had. This said, the next step is setting up a plan to compensate for the draining effects of an illness on your system.

First, learn to pace yourself throughout the day. Draw up a list of what you need to get done on a given day. Then tackle the first item on your list. When you have finished, stop and give yourself a rest period. Then tackle the next item on your list. The size and difficulty of the task will determine just how long you need to rest afterward. It will take some time to figure out how much you can do in a day. That's fine because this is a period of adjustment. You are adjusting emotionally and physically to your arthritis. You can't expect to have all the answers worked out in the first few weeks, or even months. And remember to be flexible. Some days you will feel the fatigue more than others, and will need more or longer rest periods. With a flexible schedule, you can adjust your routine as the week progresses. This brings us to the next step.

Second, establish your priorities. If you were in an office and your boss stopped by to give you a rush order, what would you do? Jump right on it and get the order out, right? But if you had four other projects sitting on your desk and all of them had *rush* written on them, you would have to decide what was your top priority. Perhaps two of them could be done by a coworker. Another two you could put off for a day or more. And the one your boss hand delivered would get the top priority. You can handle your daily chores the same way. You can get to the number-one project on your list first when you have the strength at the start of the day. Or perhaps you will choose the item which gives you the most satisfaction and accomplish it first. Then take a look at the other items and decide whether others could help you out, or would even prefer to do it themselves. Next, decide whether every task really needs to be done and weed out the unnecessary ones. Suddenly your list of chores has become more manageable.

Third, you shouldn't be reluctant to speak up when you are tired or simply can't do something yourself. Don't feel guilty or embarrassed. Accept the fact that there are certain limitations you have to live with now. Don't push yourself to the point of exhaustion or injury. And remember that people who care about you don't want you to do the impossible and hurt yourself.

Finally, take a look at all the self-help tips coming up in the next chapter. They come from people with arthritis, doctors, therapists, and trained professionals, all of whom have discovered ingenious and simple ways to get around the roadblocks and physical limitations that arthritis can throw up. Look at all the gadgets and techniques that can help you overcome the physical limitations of your condition.

Your Love Life

Everyone has experienced the nurturing and therapeutic aspects of love. Whether you are giving love or receiving it, love is food for the soul and the body. Motherly love, romantic love, the love of friendship, and the love of life all nourish us in critical ways. For someone with an illness, love is all the more important: As you go through the process of adapting to arthritis it can be essential to know that this crucial part of your life is not changing as well. The changes which come with arthritis are made easier if the quality of love in your life remains constant. This is easier said than done.

To begin with, your self-image is different. If you are a person who likes to feel in control, you may be fearful or angry because of the changes in your body as a result of arthritis or the medications you take. Even if you have always enjoyed being more dependent than independent, you may resent relying on others now because it isn't a question of choice anymore, but one of necessity. Another part of your self-image concerns your body. For better or worse, our bodies are our *own.* They are singly, individually, uniquely us, with each imperfection and attribute. Arthritis can cause changes in the joints and other parts of the body. These changes can alter the way you look, walk, sit, or gesture. They can also alter the way we see ourselves, as well as how others see us. It is going to take some hard work to learn to accept these differences in yourself. The work is made easier through the love of those around you.

Discomfort and pain will also affect how you feel about yourself. You probably don't feel attractive when you don't feel well. You may not feel strong and supportive when you are overtired. And sex may be the furthest thing from your mind when your back aches or your knees are inflamed. Let's face it, your image of yourself is going to go through a series of changes if you have arthritis. While in some ways you *are* different, in all the essential ways you are also just the same as before. You are the same person, friend, lover, grandparent, employer, parent, spouse. You are not a shadow of your former self, you are the same person with a few alterations.

Now let's look at how to restore your self-image and remain a loving and loved person. To begin, talk about the fears, angers, frustrations and annoyances that are close to your heart. For instance, tell your friends it's all right to give you a hearty hug when they see you, that you won't collapse from some loving contact. By the same token, if you are having a flare-up of inflammation or pain, warn people off—gently—before they embrace you. Save them the shock and dismay of hurting you. If your condition precludes strong physical contact, substitute equally loving and intimate gestures such as touching someone's cheek or hand. There are endless ways to physically demonstrate love and affection for friends, lovers, children, and family. Figuring them all out can be like creating a new and intimate language.

Express your frustrations. If you get upset because you can't do all the things you want to, when you want to, say so. You may be surprised to feel the tension leave the room. Maybe your children were beginning to think you really enjoyed all the extra attention and help. Maybe your wife was starting to believe that you didn't do things together as often because you didn't love her as much as you used to. Express your anger when you feel you have to. You may be angry at your arthritis for influencing your relationship with your family. Your children might need a chance to say they are angry, too—not at you but at your illness. Get it all out, because these feelings can interfere with how you relate to and show your love for your family. And these emotions can also throw up roadblocks which prevent your family and friends from showing their love and affection.

The next step you can take is to examine the problems which aren't solved simply by talking them out, then work together to find a solution or plan of action. For instance, if your children feel that you haven't been spending enough time with them, and you are feeling guilty about neglecting them, figure out a plan to correct the problem. Perhaps there is a time of day when you feel better than at other times. If you are at your best in the early afternoon, make that your special time with your children so you can be close to them and listen to their problems or personal accomplishments of the day. Weekends could be the perfect time for everyone to get special attention: There are more people home to help with chores; certain weekly tasks can be put aside for these two days; you can get out of bed later or take an afternoon nap to get some extra rest; and the hours left over for your family can be less hurried and tiring.

If you aren't married, socializing with your friends will be an important part of your life. After all, your friends are your support group, your "other" family, the people you love and who love you back. Yet if you aren't feeling well, getting up and out of the house or apartment you live in can be a big problem. On the one hand, you get depressed and lonely staying at home; on the other hand, going out is a trial at times. Again you need to plan ahead. If being around strangers in a restaurant bothers you, then tell your friends that at the moment you would like to stay away from public places and eat at someone's home. You can bring the dessert or wine if pitching in with the dinner preparations is important to you.

If you feel the changes in your body are making you uncomfortable, wear clothing you feel attractive in, or buy some new clothes which camouflage your swollen knees or elbows. If you worry about the inaccessibility of the facilities in public places, call ahead to find out if the accommodations available meet your personal physical needs. When you are dealing with close personal friends, be sure to communicate with them about the problems and uncertainties arising from your illness. Include them in the preparations for going out together. Let them participate in the planning of an afternoon's shopping expedition. It will help your friends understand your adaptation process and help them to be involved in your life. The point is that you need the support and love of the people you care about, and they continue to need yours. If you cut yourself off from your friends and your emotional needs, it will work against your mental and physical well-being.

Sexuality

Whether you are married or single, your sex life will probably be influenced by your arthritis. Consider for a moment some of the many events in life which have an effect on sex and intimacy: conflict between you and your partner; fatigue because of your work load; tension and anxiety over finances; jealousy; lack of communication; anger; interference from in-laws; misunderstandings; and competitiveness. These are just a few of the factors which can have an impact on sex and loving. Illness is another. If you have a bad cold, or even if you have had surgery or a prolonged illness, you and your loved one can usually look to the future and anticipate an eventual return to normal love relations. You can experience a temporary cessation of sex and intimacy without feeling unduly worried or threatened.

If you have arthritis, and your symptoms are more or less constant, or you have flares and remissions, the resumption of your love life can be more complicated. As we mentioned earlier, the person with arthritis has an altered self-image. You may be physically changed. You are certainly going through a variety of emotional changes as you adjust to your illness. You can have pain, discomfort, and general fatigue. You can be tense and irritable as a result of these changes. You may also be angry or depressed. Your partner is going through many of these changes as well. And the result can often be a disruption of the normal patterns of expressing your love for one another. Often, just when you need the comfort and reassurance of intimacy most, obstacles may appear. They can be overcome.

Two of the most critical factors in resuming or maintaining a close, intimate and loving relationship are communication and motivation. It may sound like a broken record, but you have got to talk to your loved one. That goes for both of you. And it is not only necessary to talk about how you feel emotionally, you also need to express how you feel physically.

Let's establish the facts up front: First of all, arthritis *almost never* directly affects the sexual parts of the body. Secondly, arthritis has no direct effect on your capacity for sexual enjoyment.

Yet there can obviously be physical problems. Pain, swelling, soreness, fatigue, changes in the way your body moves, visual changes in your body which alter your self-image, and the effects of medications are all physical aspects of the different forms of arthritis. Everyone is different and will experience these problems to different degrees.

The individual problems you confront can cause awkwardness and a decreased interest in sex. Often you can find solutions to these problems between the two of you. If you can't, or find you want some professional advice, there are doctors, nurses, and counselors who can help you. And don't forget the support and help that other people with arthritis can provide. Here are just a few of the suggestions you may find helpful:

- If your partner is hurting you, say so. And be sure to also speak up when something is giving you pleasure.
- Be creative in your sex life. If certain positions and situations are not comfortable, try out new ones until you find what is most suitable for both of you.

- Use pillows to cushion sore spots.
- Plan your sex life according to when you feel best.
- Relax with a warm shower or bath.
- Don't get overly tired if you are planning an intimate encounter.
- Do exercises to relax your joints.
- Remember that you can enjoy sensuality and affection even if you have some discomfort.

The Arthritis Foundation has published a special pamphlet called "Living and Loving with Arthritis," which discusses with sensitivity and practicality sex, intimacy, and arthritis. If sex becomes a problem, seek counseling from a social worker or health counselor without delay. Ignoring sexual concerns can only increase anxiety.

Your motivation plays an all-important role in your sex life. How much interest you have in re-establishing or maintaining a close, intimate relationship with your spouse or loved one is more significant than your physical abilities. Whether sex and intimacy represent an emotional bond or a more physical one, your willingness to fulfill your partner's and your own needs can be the determining factor.

As we have said before, physical changes can diminish your interest in sex and loving, and your self-image can be altered by an illness. If you feel less attractive or more vulnerable you may react by withdrawing from your partner. Or you may seek more frequent demonstrations of love and affection because you need the support and comfort of knowing that this aspect of your life has not changed. Another side to this is understanding what your partner and loved one needs. While you may be less interested in your sex life, your partner may feel differently. This can be an opportunity for you to remove yourself from your own concerns to concentrate on your partner's.

As we have said repeatedly, the process of accepting an illness can be a complicated and prolonged period of adjustment. Yet, any change gives us a new perspective, a new set of priorities, or goals, a chance to reflect on the past as much as on the future. Change can provide us with an opportunity to re-evaluate, to change old habits and perceptions, and to discover new things about ourselves. Rediscovering or redefining your love for the people closest to your heart can bring tremendous benefits. If the interest is there, if you are truly motivated, and if you have the help you need to overcome the uncertainties, the quality of your love life can broaden, deepen, change, and be better than ever.

Stress

Everyone is under stress. We know it, we react to it, and we try to lessen it if we can. Whether it is money, your job, hostilities at home, or simply the weather, stress affects the way we feel. The stress of an illness such as arthritis needs to be discussed further. We have mentioned already the emotional stresses of change, anger, frustration, and so forth. We have looked at the stress from fatigue and pain. Now let's examine some of the signs of stress, how they affect your arthritis, and what to do about them.

Stress symptoms can include increased pain, changes in eating habits, trouble sleeping, tight muscles, problems with concentration, and feelings of anxiety and tension. The number of stress symptoms differs from person to person, as does the degree to which they are felt. When you recognize that you are under a great deal of stress, the normal reaction is to try to reduce the stress.

Take stock of what the stresses in your life are. Then evaluate them carefully. Decide whether you can do something to eliminate the source of the stress, or whether you have to learn to live with it effectively. For example, you cannot get rid of your arthritis, thus you need to live with it as best as you can. You can get rid of some of the feelings of anger and frustration about your illness by accepting that all the anger in the world isn't going to make it go away—and it can even aggravate your disease. Don't waste your energy fighting something you won't conquer. Put your energy into coping with the aspects of your condition that you can change, such as sticking with your treatment program of exercise, medication, and rest and relaxation.

Here are some other general tips for stress management:

- Have reasonable ideas about what you can expect from yourself and others. For example, don't set the same daily goals for yourself as you did before you had arthritis because you can't expect to accomplish the same things at the same speed, with the same degree of efficiency.
- Take one day at a time and try to do something

each day that gives you pleasure, a sense of achievement, or satisfaction. Don't think about not being able to paint the kitchen by yourself. Instead, focus on planning a particularly wonderful Halloween costume for your daughter this year, or starting a local arthritis club with some of your friends.

- Improve the lines of communication with people you care about, and learn to say no without feeling guilty.
- Set about simplifying your life. Weed out the chores and activities you don't have to do so that you can concentrate on accomplishing what's important to you and your family or friends.
- Plan a daily exercise period (with the advice of your doctor). It changes the pace of your day and can play a positive part in your therapy.
- Practice a relaxation technique to reduce some of the stress built into your life. You can learn how to reduce your mental and physical tension.

Controlling Tension

Experts have developed several steps a person can take to reduce tension and bracing (the tensing-up of muscles):

- Look for telltale signs of bracing: grinding teeth, locked jaw muscles, tense neck muscles. One of the biggest clues to bracing is if you're prone to prolonged sighs. Tense neck and chest muscles disrupt your breathing. You literally hold your breath and, finally, you give out a big, long sigh.
- If you think you're a bracer, take self-help action

your attitude. Question your motives, your success." Are you pushing yourself harder eally have to? See if you can ease up on driving yourself too hard.

• When you find yourself getting tense, take an exercise break. If you're in the office, try some stretching exercises.

The key to relieving tension and bracing is relaxation. As soon as you find yourself bracing, take the following steps:

1. Retreat to a quiet room. If you're at the office, find the quietest spot you can—even the bathroom if necessary. Keep the lights as dim as possible.
2. Close your eyes. Take a deep breath. Hold for a count of two. Release your breath. Count to two. Continue to breathe deeply in this way. Inhale . . . one, two; exhale . . . one, two. Concentrate on your breathing, not your tension.
3. Tense your upper arms and shoulders. Count to five then release the muscles. Repeat at least ten times, or until you find yourself more relaxed.
4. Concentrate on your breathing again. Each time you inhale, say to yourself the word "calm." Each time you exhale, say to yourself the word "down."

Now return to what you were doing. Whenever you feel yourself bracing again during the course of the day, just begin breathing deeply and regularly and repeat to yourself, "calm down." Generally, you will indeed calm down and remove some of the stress in your daily life.

The entire exercise should not last more than five minutes, and its soothing aftereffects should last for hours.

Stress, depression, and pain are all closely related. Too much stress can cause headaches in some people, stomachaches in others, and back spasms in still others. It isn't surprising that stress can aggravate the pain associated with arthritic joints. Imagine the effect of muscles tensing from stress and pulling on an inflamed area—it hurts! Pain can also make people feel depressed sometimes. So can unrelieved stress. Depression can also have an effect on pain. When you are feeling depressed, even stubbing your toe can make you cry. And when you have painful joints, depression can make them seem to hurt more.

Just as everyone is under stress in life, so does everyone experience bouts of depression. We get depressed when a loved one dies, over bad test scores, bad news, disappointments, no-win situations, wars, other people's good luck, our own bad luck—all sorts of big and small things in life. And generally it goes away. It is only natural to be depressed by the diagnosis of a chronic illness. In a way, you are grieving for yourself and it is a typical response to bad news. For a while you just feel down, but as life goes on and things return to normal and you concentrate on other things, your depression usually goes away. Sometimes it can help to get out of the house and get a change of scenery. Or you can go to the movies—try a film which will make you laugh. For some more tips on how to cope with depression read on.

Dealing with Depression

In many cases you can overcome your depression all by yourself. Here are some things that you can do to brighten up your outlook in life:

• ***Try to pinpoint the exact cause of your depression.*** For example, ask yourself, "Am I depressed because I'm afraid my arthritis might affect my ability to perform my job?" Once you recognize the reasons behind your depression, you can look for ways to minimize the problem. Perhaps you can adapt your job slightly, discover ways to perform your everyday tasks without putting stress or strain on your arthritic joints.

In the "Simple Gadgets" section (see p. 141) you will learn about devices that can help arthritis victims cope more effectively with everyday tasks. These gadgets, used in combination with a little imagination and ingenuity, and the advice of a doctor or therapist, can help overcome many of the problems caused by stiff, painful joints. Think about how you can apply them in your job and other daily activities.

• ***Act as if you aren't depressed.*** Don't give in to your unhappiness. Even if you're feeling blue, get out of bed, get dressed, comb your hair, put on makeup or shave. Then get out of the house—even if it's just to walk next door to talk to a neighbor. Giving into depression will only prolong it.

• ***Maintain your self-esteem.*** The fact that arthritis pain limits your activities doesn't diminish your worth as a human being. Maybe you can't bowl, but you can go down to the bowling lanes with friends to talk, watch, or even keep score.

- ***Do chores on a priority basis.*** Break tasks down into small components so they don't seem overwhelming to you and trigger depression.
- ***Maintain a realistically positive attitude.*** Instead of saying, "The house is a mess and I'll never be able to clean it," divide the work into manageable portions. Tell yourself, "The house is a mess, but the kitchen is the worst, and what's really bad about the kitchen is the messy table, so first I'll clean the table." Performing this one simple chore can give you a mood-brightening sense of accomplishment.
- ***Exercise daily.*** It's one of the best ways to beat depression, and it's good for your arthritis. See the exercise section (pp. 83–90) for tips on an exercise routine designed for arthritis sufferers.
- ***Remember that you aren't alone.*** Everyone gets depressed sometimes. And it's normal for you to be frustrated and upset by arthritis pain or decreased mobility. It makes your life more difficult. But remember that the word is "difficult" not "impossible." There is still a lot you can do.

Even people with rare crippling arthritis can still talk with friends, contribute valuable ideas to business associates, and give children the benefit of their love and past experience.

If you need to talk to someone about your concerns regarding your condition, call your local Arthritis Foundation. The people there are experienced in listening to problems like yours and offering sound suggestions. Counseling can be extremely valuable in helping you to cope with even the most traumatic aspects of crippling arthritis, ranging from the inability to climb stairs or dress yourself, to the painful emotional turmoil you experience. Health care professionals have helped hundreds of people deal with these problems—they can help you, too.

A Profile in Courage

Battling swollen, pain-racked joints, Lynn Adams fought her way to the top of the women's professional racquetball circuit—and now she earns an incredible $75,000 a year at the sport!

The courageous twenty-seven-year-old overcame the agonizing problems of rheumatoid arthritis to become the Women's World Racquetball Champion.

"Sometimes my hands are so swollen and pain-racked I can't even hold my racquet—yet I refuse to let arthritis beat me," says Lynn, who's an official spokeswoman for the Arthritis Foundation.

Lynn, now married to a racquetball instructor, first learned she had the disease ten years ago. "I was crazy about athletics," she remembered. "I ran track and worked out every day. I was in peak physical condition." But rheumatoid arthritis "came like a bolt from the blue. One day my hand suddenly became hard and swollen, so painful I thought I'd broken my wrist."

The pain went away—only to return again two months later in her knee. That's when a doctor told Lynn the bad news: She had rheumatoid arthritis.

"The disease soon came in a pattern," said Lynn. "About once a month without warning it hits in a different area of my body—my hands, thighs, knees, shoulders, ankles, feet, or elbows. The pain lasts two or three days."

The disease, said Lynn, sometimes strikes at the worst possible time. Once the arthritis flared up during a four-day pro tournament. "On the third day, my right playing hand and wrist were swollen, hard and painful with arthritis," she said. "I took my medication, gritted my teeth and said to myself, 'Girl, you're gonna play!'

"I did . . . and I wasn't beaten until the finals!"

Arthritis sufferers have two battlefields on which they must beat their disease—mental and physical, according to Lynn.

"First, you can conquer the mental battleground by counting your blessings. I think of all the wonderfully courageous people who have more problems than I do—people confined to wheelchairs, iron lungs, hospital beds, people with cancer, soldiers who have lost limbs."

You can conquer the physical battlefield by keeping yourself in shape. "You can start," Lynn added, "by walking. Gradually build up until you can walk longer distances. Start an exercise program—even in your own home." And later on, if you are up to it, you can advance to mild forms of popular exercises like swimming.

"I have one other tip: When my arthritis flares up in my legs, I sit, I sew, and I do craftwork. When it flares in my racquet hand, I concentrate on other keep-fit activities."

Peter Mathon, spokesman for the Arthritis Foundation, added: "Lynn Adams is a profile in courage. She is a walking example of how a person can overcome rheumatoid arthritis to rise to the very top of professional sports."

Simple Ways to Help a Friend

Even if you don't have arthritis yourself, you can play a part in the treatment of the disease. It is really a simple role. And it can be a crucial one. If you have a little compassion, mixed in with concern, you are the perfect candidate. You can be a friend to a fellow human being.

Here are some simple tips:

- Become informed by taking the time to learn about arthritis—your friend will appreciate your interest.
- Never talk down to a person who has arthritis. A physical handicap is not a sign of any weakness.
- Be understanding about your friend's condition, but don't pity him. Pity will only make him uncomfortable and self-conscious.
- If you're going somewhere with a person who has arthritis, call ahead to make sure that when you arrive at your destination, everything will be arranged to meet his needs or disabilities.
- Don't force anyone with arthritis into activities that push him beyond his physical limitations.
- Remember that people with arthritis have good and bad days. The quality of these days are not within their control, so be ready to adjust your plans to fit their needs at a particular moment.
- Don't try to give medical advice to someone with arthritis or steer him or her toward some "new miracle treatment." Quack remedies do little but raise false hopes and empty your wallet.
- If you're in doubt about how to act in a certain situation with a person who has arthritis, put yourself in

his place. Ask yourself, "If I were he, would I want someone to do that?"

• If you have children who are going to be meeting someone with arthritis, prepare the children in advance. Explain that arthritis is a disease that can force someone to walk slowly, confine the individual to a wheelchair, or even deform him. Tell children that they should not treat someone with arthritis any differently than other people, nor should they offer any comments about the disability.

Juvenile Rheumatoid Arthritis (JRA) and Its Emotional Effects

The chronic illness of a loved one is a heavy emotional burden for a family to bear, especially when that person is a child. Normal family life can be disrupted, and all the members of the family may experience some troubling emotions. It is essential to deal with these feelings in order to cope with the disease.

Typically, when parents learn that their child has arthritis, they experience feelings of shock, numbness, and disbelief. As the child begins receiving treatment, other children in the family may feel rejected because of the amount of time and attention their ill sibling is receiving from their parents. Sometimes the other children feel guilty, as if they were somehow responsible for their brother or sister's illness.

The parents often feel guilty, too, wondering if there was something they could have done to prevent the disease from developing.

Arthritis is difficult enough for an adult to accept, so imagine how difficult it can be for a child. The child with arthritis may experience many conflicting and painful emotions. The child with JRA may feel that the painful condition is some sort of punishment; blame his parents for the illness; adopt a self-pitying "why me?" attitude; or indulge in anger because he can't be as active as he was before. He may also resent healthy children who can play and do things he can't—including his brothers and sisters.

It is essential for the JRA patient and his family to discuss their feelings openly in order to restore a normal and healthy atmosphere to their household. As the parent of a child with JRA, how do you and your spouse honestly feel about your child's illness? How do you think you can help him cope with it? How do you think your other children feel about it? How can you help them to cope with their sibling's illness? How can you help all of your children develop a positive attitude regarding the limitations imposed by arthritis? There's no point in pretending nothing is wrong and that your lives can go on exactly as they did before. Arthritis is a new part of your family and should be dealt with openly and honestly.

Sometimes it is difficult for someone with JRA to discuss his feelings. The best way to encourage him to express himself is for the parents to first discuss their own feelings with him. If the parents "go first," it may be easier for the child to talk about his problems and concerns. Once the child does speak up, you will probably be pleasantly surprised at his ability to cope with the disease. Be prepared, though, for the possibility that he may express anger at your powerlessness to spare him from undergoing painful tests and for your role in limiting his activities. You can help your child by allowing open expressions of anger from time to time. He has a right to be frustrated and angry, but don't let his anger become continuous or uncontrolled. Then a child may even express his resentment by refusing to take his medication or do his exercises. If his anger seems excessive or out-of-control, you should seek counseling.

As a parent, you can also monitor and guide the behavior of other members of your family. Discourage your other children from treating the JRA child with excessive sympathy, pity, or forced cheerfulness. Any of these can make a child with JRA uncomfortable, different, and bitter.

The normal relationships between husband and wife and between parents and children may have to be temporarily set aside during the early stages of a child's illness. However, you should make every effort to permit the entire family to spend special times together. You should also let your other children know that you understand they might be feeling a little neglected, and explain to them that it's just a temporary situation. Once the family adjusts emotionally to arthritis, things will calm down and resentments should fade.

You can expect changes in your own feelings and attitudes as time progresses. What may have at first seemed an impossible situation will gradually become manageable as the disease is brought under control and your child shows signs of improvement.

Growing Up with Arthritis

Most children with arthritis grow into adulthood without any significant physical disability. It's important that they reach adulthood equally free of any emotional disabilities.

The child with JRA may be physically smaller and slower to mature sexually than other children. He may tire easily, have trouble keeping up with playmates, and be unable to participate in some activities with other children. Without meaning to, other children and adults can make these situations even more difficult by treating the arthritic child as someone "special." Being "special" can be upsetting, especially during the teen-age years when being just like other kids is important.

Some children will need extra encouragement to help them deal effectively with their condition. Additional reassurance can be especially valuable if the child is in pain and is fearful that any physical activity may increase his pain. Gentle encouragement may also offset some JRA victim's tendency to use their illness as an excuse to avoid household chores and responsibilities.

The attitudes held by the parents of a child with JRA strongly affect the child's feelings about himself and his condition. While it's only natural for a parent to try to protect a child with a disability, there is the risk of making your child too dependent if you do everything for him or if you completely excuse him from household tasks. If you expect nothing from the child, he may begin to feel useless and unproductive. Children with arthritis can do many things for themselves, and encouraging them to be as self-sufficient as possible will make them feel better about themselves. Appropriate and continuing encouragement will require time and patience from both the parents and their child.

Children with arthritis should also try to learn and understand as much as they can about their disease and treatment. An older child can reasonably be expected to take responsibility for taking medication, reporting side effects, and following an exercise program.

Establishing a routine can be the key to helping a young person with JRA adjust to his condition. The presence of the disease itself may make a child feel as if his life has gone out of control—adhering to a schedule of exercise periods, rest periods, doctor visits, and so forth, can reassure your child that he is still in control.

CHAPTER VIII

Self-Help Tips

IT IS EASY TO FORGET THAT IN ADDITION TO EVERYthing medicine can do to help the arthritis patient, he can and should help himself. Sometimes it is tempting to just say, "It's the doctor's job to help me, that's what he's trained to do!" and leave it at that. But then we have given up all control over our own destiny. Instead, the arthritis sufferer should make a pact with himself and his doctor, to share the responsibility for getting better. It takes a sense of personal responsibility to make yourself do your exercises. It also takes responsibility to protect your joints and prevent further unnecessary damage.

No one is asking you to be a doctor—that's not your job. But you should learn about the simple, commonsense approaches to protecting your body, and reducing the pain of everyday activities from getting dressed to preparing a meal. This approach is fully endorsed by the Arthritis Foundation which says, "You will look happier, sleep better, have better mobility and a better mental outlook on your disease. You will feel like you have taken control of your life again." These are the objectives of the self-help therapy. If you follow this commonsense plan you can expect to reduce your pain and live a more normal life.

Reduce Stress on Your Joints

• Always try to use the strongest or largest joint possible to perform any task in order to relieve the strain on smaller joints. For example, use your entire hand to push cupboard doors closed instead of using just your fingers.

• Instead of using your hand or arm to close a drawer, try using your hip. This distributes physical stress over the largest area possible.

• Try not to use your fingers or hand to push down on the lid of a plastic container—use your elbow.

• When using a spray or pump bottle, try pushing down with the palm of your hand instead of the top of your finger.

• Whenever you can, consider distributing the load over several joints. For example, instead of lifting a coffee cup with one hand, use both hands.

• You have to try to avoid keeping joints in the same position for any length of time. Arthritic joints tend to stiffen when they're still, and this can cause more pain when they're finally moved. If you're holding something, say the telephone, take frequent breaks to stretch and move your fingers.

• Similarly, when you sit down for a long time, try to get up and stretch once in a while. When rising from a chair, push yourself forward to the edge of the seat.

Place one foot slightly ahead of the other. Then lean forward until your hips automatically start to rise off the chair.

• Remember to take breaks between tasks and try to conserve your energy. Don't feel you have to complete big jobs all at once. Do what is most important first, plan ahead, and get help when you need it. Stop and rest before you become overtired.

• Try to learn to respect pain—and know when pain is a signal to stop whatever you're doing. A good general rule is that if an activity causes a joint to become painful, and the pain endures for more than a few hours—then that particular activity is harmful. Don't do it again.

Arthritis-Proof Your Kitchen

• To avoid stress on your hands and fingers, you might want to consider having straps looped on your refrigerator and cupboard doors. Then you can open them with your forearm by placing your arm through the strap and pulling.

• When opening cans, use an electric can opener or a wall-mounted manually-operated opener. Hand-held openers can be extremely painful to operate.

• Open a flip-top can by inserting a knife under the metal tab and using the knife as a lever.

• Try to use lightweight appliances. Buy the lightest possible vacuum cleaner. Buy garbage cans with wheels so you don't have to lift them. Use shopping carts not only in the grocery store, but for any shopping.

• Instead of scouring pads, try getting a wire brush scourer with a handle to clean pots and pans.

• When beating eggs or other foods, it's useful to remember that a whisk offers less physical resistance than a fork or spoon.

• Install single-lever faucets in your kitchen, bath, or laundry room. They're easier to manage than the dual hot and cold knobs that require a strong twist to turn on and off.

• Open jars with your palms instead of your fingers. Simply place the jar on a table and put your palm over the top of the lid. Lean forward, apply pressure to the lid and turn your palm while holding the jar with your other hand.

• Try to use utensils that have fat wooden handles. If you have problems grasping a handle, try padding it with a towel or foam rubber.

• Make sure your cutting tools and kitchen knives are sharp. They require less pressure to cut and are less likely to slip if they are sharp.

• Consider rearranging your storage system for tools and kitchen utensils so that the items you use most frequently are close at hand.

Arthritis-Proof Your Bathroom

• Install extenders on toilet seats. These extenders will raise the seat four or more inches and reduce stress on your hips and legs whenever you sit down or get up.

• Try using nonskid rubber mats in the bath and

shower and on the floor where you stand to get in and out of the tub. Sturdy grab bars will also make it easier to get in and out of the tub.

• When taking a bath or shower, put the soap in a cloth bag or on a string around your neck, because dropped soap can be painful to retrieve. A bath mitt can help in scrubbing.

Arthritis-Proof Your Wardrobe

To an arthritis victim, the simple act of getting dressed can be a painful ordeal. Specially made clothing can ease the pain of getting dressed.

Some mail-order firms offer garments that slip on and off easily and can be fastened or unfastened without buttons and zippers.

In place of buttons, which can be extremely difficult for arthritis victims with stiff fingers to manipulate, these clothes feature wraparound closures and easy-to-handle Velcro fasteners concealed behind mock buttons.

You can also make your wardrobe easier to manage by getting rid of clothes that need ironing, and replacing them with garments made of permanent-press fabrics. Choose clothes with front openings whenever possible. This can be expensive if you try to replace your wardrobe all at once, but over a period of several years you can gradually adapt your clothes to your physical limitations.

Dr. James Fries, Director of the Stanford University Arthritis Clinic, also has some clothing tips to offer:

• Select clothes that are easy to put on such as slip-on shoes, wraparound robes, clip-on ties, and stretch belts that hook rather than fasten.

• Use a long-handled shoe horn, and for help putting on socks, use garter snaps or clothespins wrapped in tape.

• Get a valet stand to hold your shirt while you put it on.

• Use a dresser made of lightweight wood with small, well-lubricated drawers, and replace small knobs with big handles.

• Do not wear shoes with pointed toes and avoid high heels—they throw additional weight on the forefoot and can cause foot pain.

• To eliminate pain in the ball of the foot, have a shoemaker put a *metatarsal bar*—an extra strip of leather—on the outside of the sole an inch behind where the weight is usually borne.

• Pain in the heel can be eased considerably by using a shoe with a high wedge and a lot of padding, which limits the stretch on the Achilles' tendon. Also consider elastic shoelaces that can be left in place at a comfortable tension.

Simple Gadgets to Ease Arthritis Pain

1. *Dressing*. Simple sticks with hooks on the ends are helpful for putting on shoes and stockings. There are also U-shaped stocking aids that allow you to put on hose without bending over.

2. *Rising*. "Often people with arthritis have trouble getting up from a sitting position because the seats are

too low," says Dr. Eric P. Gall, associate professor of internal medicine in rheumatology at the University of Arizona College of Medicine.

Dr. Gall suggests raising your favorite chair a few inches by placing it on a platform, or using barstool-type chairs to ease the pain of getting in and out of low chairs.

People with arthritis can also reduce the pain they suffer getting in and out of chairs by using remarkable new chair elevators called Pedi-4-Legs. The elevators attach to chair legs, and can raise the rear of the chair to make getting up easier and less painful.

Pedi-4-Legs, which are small enough to take along on trips, are available at hospital and surgical supply stores.

3. *Reaching.* The most common reaching gadgets available are long-handled tongs, fifteen to thirty inches long, that allow you to pull items down from a shelf or to turn food in a low broiler.

4. *Gripping.* It's easier to grasp things such as knives, forks, or spoons when you increase the width of the handles with foam rubber, cloth, or other materials. Self-help outlets sell grip-widening gadgets.

5. *Turning.* You can buy adapters that fit over doorknobs, enabling you to simply press a handle to open a door instead of having to fumble with the round, hard-to-grasp knob. Similar devices include extensions that fit over faucet handles to give you more leverage in turning them on and off.

Says Dr. Gall: "Self-help gadgets can ease the pain and help protect the joints—especially when they eliminate needlessly repetitive tasks."

For information on how to obtain these and similar

devices, contact your local chapter of the Arthritis Foundation for its self-help manual.

10 Tips to Help You Sleep

Sleepiness can plague anyone. Often it makes you feel that you can't cope with the trials—or enjoy the rewards—of the next day because you aren't at your best. It should come as no surprise that pain often keeps arthritis sufferers awake at night—but following these ten simple tips can result in a good night's sleep.

1. *Try twin beds* if you have a restless partner who keeps you awake at night. If your bedmate tosses and turns, forcing you frequently to shift positions, the discomfort that results can trigger the sharp painful twinges that disrupt sleep.

2. *Sleep on a moderately firm mattress.* This allows the easiest, least painful movement. Water beds have worked well for some people. Before you choose, it is best to test a number of mattresses to determine which is best for comfortable body repositioning.

3. *Place your pillows in strategic positions* to limit painful body movement. Position the pillows to cushion yourself against any turning. One caution: If your arthritis affects your knees or hips, refrain from placing pillows under your knees. A stiff, bent joint may result.

4. *Consider a nightcap*—it may help. Drinking alcoholic beverages is an individual decision, but many people feel that a simple glass of wine, or no more than an ounce of hard liquor, helps them relax and sleep.

Inventive Arthritis Sufferer

When arthritis forced her into a wheelchair, courageous Elmora Simms worked hard to find some simple ways of making housework easier and less painful. "A lot of these tips came from trial and error, and most of the errors were painful," said Mrs. Simms of Columbus, Ohio. "But now I have worked out a good system of helpful hints to get arthritis sufferers through life."

Up until 1964, Mrs. Simms worked as a casket trimmer doing detailed sewing. When she was struck by rheumatoid arthritis she had to stop working. Eventually, after she was confined to a wheelchair and had lost her husband, Mrs. Simms found herself confronted with the impossible—fending for herself when she couldn't even walk!

"Your life can't stop because of arthritis. You have to keep going. You can't imagine how frustrating it is to try to open a jar when your fingers can't grip the lid. I broke into tears one day because I was so frustrated with a bottle that I couldn't open.

"It took quite awhile to learn all the tricks, but with the help of family and friends, and reading a lot, I managed to collect a lot of tips that make housekeeping and taking care of the family a lot easier."

In the kitchen, Mrs. Simms suggests taking round sponge protectors from electric hair curlers and slipping them over the handles of knives, forks and spoons to make handling easier. "And keep a pair of long-handled tongs around. If you drop something, it's a lot easier to pick it up with the tongs.

Shares Tips to Ease Housework

"It may sound strange, but a pair of pliers can be very handy. You can open a milk carton or just about anything with them. Pliers are also good for turning small knobs—such as the timer clock on the stove.

"Clothespins are good for sealing bags that come with those hard-to-handle wire twists. If you have kitchen cupboards with magnetic locks, putting a piece of scotch tape on the magnetic surface will make them open more easily.

"Keep a beer can opener handy for prying lids off plastic containers. Buy salt and pepper shakers that have handles; there is nothing worse than having them slip out of your grip and into the stew. Buy coffee cups with handles that have holes for two fingers. To carry small items from the kitchen to the dining room table, put them in a large container with handles.

"Keep a hammer and knife handy for tough cutting jobs. If you want to cut through cabbage or a potato, for example, just place the knife on top of the cabbage and tap the blade through with the hammer.

"Shape a clothespin to fit the dial holes on your telephone. It makes it far easier to dial if you have arthritic hands or fingers.

"Here's a recreational tip. If you like jigsaw puzzles, put a piece of double-sided tape on your fingers and you'll be able to pick up the pieces like magic. The tape also helps turn the pages of newspapers and magazines."

alcohol can harm the quality of your ... ur health.

... a pre-bedtime exercise routine. Exercise ... stiffness and pain from developing in joints, and it's an excellent way to unwind. Sex before going to sleep is a great idea.

6. *Try a warm bath.* Thirty minutes in a warm tub can reduce muscle tension and induce the drowsiness that precedes restful sleep.

7. *Stay away from sleeping pills and sedatives.* They do not provide deep, restful sleep—and if used too often, they can result in drug dependency.

8. *Reschedule your anti-inflammatory drug dosage.* If your doctor has instructed you to adjust your own anti-inflammatory drug dosage, take the largest dose before bedtime.

9. *Take daytime naps.* When sleep is disrupted night after night, a cycle of sleeplessness can easily result due to intense fatigue. Three or four five-minute naps a day can take the edge off fatigue and break the cycle.

10. *Switch to loose-fitting night clothes.* The clothing you wear to bed should be comfortable. It is also advisable to use lightweight comforters and blankets.

A New Kind of Mattress Pad May Help You Sleep

A new mattress pad made from weaving wool (brand name: Woolrest) may give arthritis and back pain sufferers a good night's sleep, some experts say.

"We're not exactly sure why it works—but it works,"

said Dr. Peter Dickson, Ph.D., assistant professor of marketing at Ohio State University. He tested the Woolrest pad on 250 people in Ohio, New Zealand, and Australia. About half those tested had either arthritis or back pain.

"Over 90 percent said it increased the comfort of their bed," Dickson said. "About two-thirds said that it improved their sleep. And 40 to 60 percent of those with back pain or arthritis report that it relieved their symptoms of muscle and back pain. Tossing and turning for someone who suffers from muscle or back pain can cause very aggravated sleep," Dr. Dickson added.

"Woolrest may help people remain comfortable longer and help them stay longer in one position to maintain a very deep, relaxed sleep at night."

Sleeping Bags for Arthritis Victims

Sleeping in sleeping bags relieves morning stiffness in some arthritis patients, says a leading medical expert. After several of his patients tried the simple method, Dr. Earl Brewer said: "The results were amazing. I was quite surprised at the success I was having with some of these people."

Dr. Brewer said he had stumbled on the technique quite by accident. One of his young patients wanted to go on a camping trip, but the boy's parents were concerned. "At home the boy was always stiff in the morning, and his parents were worried that lying out on the cold ground he would be even more stiff," explained Dr. Brewer. "But the youngster went along, and when he got up in the morning he wasn't stiff at all."

Dr. Brewer, chief of rheumatology services at Texas Children's Hospital in Houston and a professor of pediatrics at Baylor College of Medicine, says sleeping bags are effective retainers of heat. The patient's body stays warmer and, as a result, the stiffness is substantially reduced.

Morning stiffness is a problem for most sufferers of arthritis, and many of them could be helped by the sleeping bag. "This is something that could be potentially helpful to a lot of people, not just children," said Dr. Brewer. But, he cautioned, "It's not curing anyone. It just helps the stiffness."

Night Gloves to Relieve Morning Pain

Millions of arthritic sufferers can get dramatic relief from nagging pain and morning stiffness in their hands—simply by wearing stretch gloves at night.

The gloves are available at many department stores and they seem to reduce the throbbing, swelling, and aching in both *rheumatoid arthritis* and *osteoarthritis* sufferers.

"What the gloves do is to keep the blood flowing in the hands the same way supportive stockings keep it flowing in the legs," explained arthritis expert Dr. George Ehrlich. "This prevents stagnation, aching, stiffness, and that numb feeling in the hands. The gloves measurably reduce throbbing as well."

There have been several studies conducted on stretch gloves. The first was conducted by Dr. Ehrlich when he was director of the arthritis center at Temple University's Albert Einstein Medical Center in Philadelphia. His subjects were forty-four *rheumatoid arthritis* and *osteoarthritis* sufferers.

Dr. Frank Schmid conducted a more recent study, funded in part by the Arthritis Foundation, on twenty-three people with *rheumatoid arthritis.* "The gloves reduced swelling, stiffness, and numbness," reported Dr. Schmid, chief of the section of arthritis-connective tissue diseases at Northwestern University Medical School.

Added Dr. Ehrlich: "Ask your doctor before you wear them. If they are uncomfortable, pull them off."

Heat and Cold Therapy

Heat treatments are a time-tested and effective way to relax muscles and alleviate joint pain and soreness. These treatments tend to be most helpful in the morning, when arthritis sufferers often feel stiff. The heat is also useful for limbering up stiff joints before exercising.

There are many ways to apply heat to a painful joint, including hot baths and showers, heat lamps (not sunlamps), electric pads, and electric mitts. Some methods may be more effective for your condition than others, so be sure to check with your doctor before you apply heat to a painful joint. Some heat methods, especially heat lamps, can be dangerous if they aren't used properly.

Some people may find cold treatments more effective in relieving pain. The use of cold compresses or ice bags wrapped in towels can help numb the affected area and reduce blood circulation so pain is not as strong or intense.

You can relieve the pain of arthritic knees with amazing ease by placing plastic bags filled with ice water on them three times a day. In a recent study at a Philadelphia hospital, this simple "kitchen cure" was used by medical researchers on twenty-four patients with arthritic knees—and they reported astonishing success.

"Every one of the twenty-four showed an improved muscle strength, freedom of movement, and increased speed in standing up," declared Dr. Peter Utsinger who headed the medical team.

"They also averaged an extra hour of sleep and cut their doses of medication in half. The therapy had no side effects," the researchers reported.

Dr. Utsinger, head of immunology at Germantown Hospital and Medical Center, explained that eleven-inch by thirteen-inch plastic bags were filled with ordinary tap water and six ice cubes. "Then," he said, "when the patients were seated comfortably with the arthritic knee extended, one ice bag was placed on top of the knee and another beneath it."

The study was conducted for four weeks, he said, with patients holding the ice packs on their knees for twenty-minute periods three times a day. Although Dr. Utsinger's study was done on *rheumatoid arthritis* patients, the method can be used by any other arthritis sufferers as well.

Diet and Nutrition

Anyone, healthy or not, should try to eat a well-rounded diet. If you are under the stress of illness, proper nutrition is even more important, because stress —whether it comes from anxiety or sickness—depletes your body's nutrients.

There is a continuing debate over the usefulness of vitamin and mineral supplements in addition to eating nutritional foods. The Arthritis Foundation states that nutrition has an important effect on your health but it warns against following "quick cure" diets which claim miraculous relief for people with any form of arthritis. It adds that since the causes of most types of arthritis have not been established as yet, unproved theories incorporating fad diets are a waste of time and money.

How Do I Get a Balanced Diet?

The conventional wisdom of the medical profession is that a balanced diet requires that you select foods from each of four basic food groups every day: meats, poultry, and fish; vegetables and fruits; milk products; and breads and cereals.

- **Meats,** including poultry and fish, supply protein, as do eggs, nuts, dried peas and beans. A three-ounce beef patty, or three ounces of chicken plus one cup of dried peas, or two eggs will meet this dietary requirement.
- **Vegetables and fruits** contain some carbohydrates, fiber and iron. Many contain vitamins A and C as well. Try to eat at least two servings from this food group

every day. It's also a good idea to eat dark green and deep yellow vegetables at least twice a week—they are an excellent source of vitamin A.

• **Milk products,** including hard cheese and yogurt, supply calcium, phosphorous (a mineral), and riboflavin (a vitamin), as well as protein. Two cups of milk or yogurt, or two ounces of cheese a day, will fulfill most adult dietary requirements.

• **Breads and cereals,** including pasta and rice, supply your body with carbohydrates, fiber, and many of the essential B vitamins. These foods also contain some protein, iron, and minerals. Four servings a day are recommended.

There is a fifth food group which contains fats, alcoholic beverages, and all those sweet, sugary, and oily snacks that are often labeled "junk food." These foods may be appealing, but they supply little besides carbohydrates. Eliminating junk food is the best way to cut down on calories.

Calories?

A calorie is a measurement of heat. Your body "burns" food, and calories are a simple way to express how much energy is available for your body to burn. When planning a healthy diet, you need to think about both calories and nutrients. Both are important, but calories are what control the weight you lose or gain. A lettuce leaf, for example, has virtually no calories, but does have some nutritional value. A piece of candy, on the other hand, supplies large amounts of calories, but has practically no nutritional value.

On Being Overweight

Overweight people develop *osteoarthritis* more frequently than do people of normal weight. Carrying excess weight over a period of years can put extra stress on weight-bearing joints such as the hips and knees. If you have arthritis, it's important to avoid placing this extra burden on your body. And because many overweight people tend to be less physically active than normal, they may also suffer from increased joint stiffness.

If you need to lose weight, cutting down on cakes, sweets, fatty meats, and soft drinks will decrease your calorie intake without depriving your body of essential nutrients. Be sure to consult your doctor before you go on a weight reduction program.

When You're Not Eating at Home

There's no need to alter your good eating habits when you dine in a restaurant. Nearly all menus offer foods that won't disrupt your diet. Simply ask your waiter to have your fish or chicken baked or steamed. Have your vegetable served plain, without butter or sauces.

When friends invite you for meals in their homes, don't hesitate to mention your dietary needs in advance. Most hosts would rather prepare something everyone can enjoy than have you neglect your food. If you feel it would be rude to mention your diet, you must be prepared to walk away from the table hungry. It's your choice.

A Checklist of DOs and DON'Ts

Here is a quick checklist of what you should and should not do if you suffer from the symptoms of arthritis. Sometimes it is easier to have a chart to refer to when you are in doubt about whether to do some activity or use some technique to help your pain. Or maybe you just want a quick review of helpful hints as you start your day. However you use this chart, remember that it is only a general guide to help you cope with the limitations of arthritis and reduce suffering.

DO . . .	DON'T . . .
. . . sit upright in a straight-back chair with a firm seat, with your feet firmly on the floor.	. . . slouch while sitting in a chair.
. . . try to sleep as much as possible lying straight, flat on your back. Keep your knees and hips straight with arms and hands straight by your side.	. . . sleep on your stomach, because this can cause neck and back pain. (The only exception—if you have arthritis of the hip, knee or back, sleep on your stomach.)
. . . use any splint, brace or other self-help aid that	. . . be too proud or embarrassed to use a crutch,

DO . . .	DON'T . . .
your doctor or therapist has prescribed for you.	cane or walker to take stress and strain off inflamed joints.
. . . use counters, tables and other furniture for support when moving around your home.	. . . lean to one side or the other when lifting yourself out of a chair or off a toilet seat. This causes dangerous twisting strains.
. . . use a 250-watt reflector heat lamp to focus heat on a single part of your body.	. . . use a sun lamp, ultraviolet light or hair dryer to heat your joints.
. . . do your exercises over several short periods each day to prevent stiffening of your joints.	. . . engage in high-tension exercises such as weight lifting, which places stress on the joints, unless specifically prescribed.
. . . take a daily twenty-minute tub bath in warm water to apply heat simultaneously to widely	. . . lie on a heating pad or fall asleep with one on your body.

DO . . .	DON'T . . .
separated joints—or take a shower if you can't get into the tub.	
. . . wear properly fitting shoes with heels that are low and wide.	. . . wear "high-style" shoes with pointed toes or platform heels.
. . . eat well-balanced nutritious meals that include vegetables, fruits, whole grains, meat and dairy products.	. . . allow yourself to get overweight because this puts an extra burden on your joints.
. . . take your full prescribed dosage of aspirin—or other anti-inflammatory drugs—even when your condition improves.	. . . rely on exotic remedies—such as green-lipped mussel extract—to cure your arthritis.

CHAPTER IX

Other Diseases Associated with Arthritis

THIS CHAPTER EXAMINES OTHER FORMS OF ARTHRItis as well as several closely related disorders. All of these conditions belong to the family of rheumatic diseases. Rheumatic diseases include those that affect the joints and those that affect the supportive tissues—tendons, ligaments and muscles—outside the joint. *Osteoarthritis* and *rheumatoid arthritis* are examples of the first group, as are *gout* and *juvenile rheumatoid arthritis*. *Fibrositis*, *tendonitis*, and *bursitis* are examples of disorders involving the supportive tissues. Rheumatic diseases can also involve other parts of the body such as the skin and internal organs. Frequently, the term *arthritis* is used to represent rheumatic diseases in general.

You can use this chapter as a layman's reference book on other common diseases associated with arthritis, but only your doctor can diagnose and treat arthritis. Perhaps this section can help you to be more understanding of people with arthritis because you will know more about what they are going through and how they feel. However you use it, this information about a condition which affects thirty-six million people is sure to surprise you.

Gout (Gouty Arthritis)

If, in the middle of the night, you suddenly wake up with a searing pain in your big toe, you may have *gout.* But it could be some time before this is confirmed by your doctor because the condition is often misdiagnosed.

Gout is a potentially crippling form of arthritis that affects more than one million Americans. But the good news is that *gout* is one of the most treatable of all the forms of chronic arthritis, according to Dr. Herbert Diamond of the Downstate Medical Center in New York.

Although *gout* can strike any joint in the body, it is most often found in the joints of the legs. At least half of all of those who have *gout* develop it at some time in the joint of the big toe.

Gout is a clear signal that some of your body's processes are out of control, resulting in a build-up of uric acid. This condition, called *hyperuricemia,* indicates that your kidneys aren't removing uric acid fast enough, or that your body is producing too much uric acid to begin with. Uric acid is a chemical made by the liver and results from the breakdown of substances called purines, which are found in all of the cells of the body as well as in most foods. They are highly concentrated in certain rich foods.

Normally uric acid circulates in your blood until it is passed into urine in the kidneys and out of your body. When you have *gout,* however, the uric acid changes into urate crystals which are deposited in joints and other tissues. An attack of *gout* occurs when these crystals get into a joint and cause irritation leading to inflammation.

What Causes Gout?

While scientists have determined that the direct cause of an acute attack of *gout* is the deposit of urate crystals in a joint, they don't yet know why or how these crystals get into joints. *Gout* can be an inherited condition, or it can occur as a complication of other ailments.

An attack of *gout* can be triggered by drinking too much alcohol or eating large amounts of food with high concentrations of purines, or by the rapid loss of tissue from crash dieting, or, occasionally, by trauma to a joint.

Who Has Gout?

Gout, the third most common form of arthritis, affects nearly two million Americans. There are ten men who get it to every one woman. Overweight men over forty who drink, according to Dr. Edward W. Holmes of the Duke University Medical Center Gout Clinic, make good targets. The few women who do develop *gout* seldom have it until after menopause. The condition is also very rare in children.

What Are the Symptoms?

An acute attack of *gout* is extremely painful. The affected joint is swollen, red, hot, and throbbing. The skin over the joint looks shiny and sometimes turns purple. The joint area may be so sensitive to touch that even the brush of a bedsheet can cause intense pain.

These acute attacks often come very quickly. *Gout* patients report that they usually go to bed feeling fine and wake up in the middle of the night in pain. At first, *gout* attacks are few and far between, and they last no longer than a few days. Then your body seems to go back to normal. However, if the disease is not controlled by medical treatment, the attacks may come more often and last longer. Repeated attacks signify that damage is occurring in the joint, which can leave your joint stiff and limited in motion even after the attack is over.

How Does a Doctor Diagnose Gout?

A doctor will ask you to describe your symptoms and then examine you. A sudden, very painful attack in only one joint, probably the big toe, clearly suggests *gout.* There are some other forms of arthritis that can act like *gout,* however. For example, *pseudogout, septic arthritis,* and even *rheumatoid arthritis* can have very similar symptoms, but they are not the result of urate crystal deposits. The only way to diagnose *gout* with certainty is for your doctor to remove fluid from the joint, examine it, and determine if urate crystals are present.

The doctor may also perform tests to measure the amount of uric acid in your blood. Remember, though, that a high level of uric acid doesn't necessarily mean you have gout. (In fact, most people with *hyperuricemia* never get attacks of *gout.*) And conversely, a low level of uric acid doesn't necessarily mean that you don't have *gout.*

A doctor will also look for urate crystal deposits in other parts of your body—appearing as lumps under the skin. These lumps can appear along the outer edge of the ear, over the elbow, or near the affected joint. If untreated, these deposits can damage other parts of the body besides the joints. These crystals can also collect in the urine, forming gravel or even stones, a condition that usually strikes people who pass too little fluid from their body. High blood pressure and kidney infections may result from *gout,* so your doctor should look for these indicators as well.

Drugs for Gout Patients

Colchicine: This prescription drug is an ancient and effective remedy for an acute attack of *gout.* It may be injected directly into your bloodstream for faster relief. The drug can cause severe diarrhea, making it necessary to stop treatment.

Benemid (probenecid): This drug makes the gout patient pass more uric acid into the urine, so that he or she will be less likely to experience an attack of *gout.* It is of no value in treating the acute attack itself, however. In fact, when a person first starts taking the drug he may have a temporary increase in attacks.

Zyloprim (allopurinol): Zyloprim cuts down on your body's production of uric acid. Inform your doctor immediately if you experience a skin rash or any other side effect.

Diet and Gout

There are many myths concerning the effect diet has on *gout*. Here are the facts:

1. If you're overweight, you should ask your doctor to recommend and supervise a weight loss program. You should not fast or try to diet too abruptly.
2. There are a few foods your doctor will tell you to avoid because they tend to raise the level of uric acid (see the *Purine Content of Common Foods* chart below). Usually people with *gout* can eat what they want in moderation, but you should discuss your normal diet thoroughly with your doctor.
3. You can drink coffee and tea. You can also drink alcohol in moderation (about two ounces of hard liquor, a can of beer, or a glass of wine a day). Drinking large amounts of alcohol can bring on an attack of *gout* in some people.
4. A high daily intake of nonalcoholic liquids is important (a minimum of two quarts is recommended), especially for those patients who have *gout* and kidney stones.

Purine Content of Common Foods

The purines found in many foods don't cause *gout* but they can bring on an attack of the condition if consumed in excessive quantities. It's best to limit your intake of foods with high purine contents if you suffer from *gout*.

Group A: Foods containing a high level of purines. Avoid these foods as much as possible.

liver	gravies
sweetbreads	broths
brains	mussels
fish roe	wine
beer	anchovies
kidney	heart
sardines	herring

Group B: Foods containing moderate amounts of purine. Limit yourself to one serving per day.

meats	mushrooms
peas	spinach
cauliflower	whole grain cereals
lentils	fowl
yeast	fish (except those above)
beans	other seafoods
asparagus	

Group C: Foods containing small amounts of purines. You can eat as much of these as you want.

vegetables (except those listed above)	refined cereals and cereal products
fruits	butters and fats (some moderation required)
milk	sugar and sweets
cheese	plain, clear
eggs	vegetable soups
spices and condiments (including salt and pepper)	nuts

Juvenile Rheumatoid Arthritis, the Children's Disease

As many as 250,000 children under the age of sixteen in the United States suffer from some form of arthritis.

Children are subject to several disorders connected with arthritis. *Ankylosing spondylitis,* which affects the spine and hips, is usually found in boys. *Systemic lupus,* which affects the joints and many internal organs, as well as the skin, is mostly a disease found in girls.

In addition, there are three forms of *Juvenile Rheumatoid Arthritis* (JRA) which can be quite serious. The signs and symptoms can vary from day to day, or even between morning and afternoon. Joint stiffness and pain can be slight one day and then so severe the next that the child can barely move without great difficulty. Fortunately, the outlook for most children is relatively good.

Each of the three forms of JRA affects the body differently and is accompanied by different signs and symptoms.

- *Systemic JRA:* The entire body, including internal organs, is affected.
- *Polyarticular JRA:* Several joints are affected. ("Poly" means several and "articular" means concerning or pertaining to joints.)
- *Pauciarticular JRA:* Only a few joints are affected. ("Pauci" means few.)

What Causes JRA?

Scientists don't know what causes any of the forms of

JRA. They do know that it is not contagious, so your child didn't catch it from someone else, and can't give it to anyone. Heredity is known to be an important factor in some instances, but its roll is still unclear. Research continues in the search for the cause of JRA. It is hoped that once the cause is found doctors may be able to cure this illness and even to prevent it before it starts.

What Are the Symptoms?

Although each form of JRA has its own individual symptoms, you should be alert to some general signs.

Inflammation is the key ingredient in every kind of *juvenile rheumatoid arthritis.* Inflammation causes pain, heat, swelling, and stiffness in your child's joints. The lining of the joint becomes swollen and overgrown, and produces excess fluid.

Since it hurts to move an inflamed joint, your child may try to keep it still. That's often not a good idea. Lack of movement for long periods leads to increased stiffness in the joint and weakness in the muscles around it. Eventually, without movement, the structure around the joint may tighten up and shorten, causing a deformity known as a *joint contracture.* Doctors usually prescribe a physical activity program to prevent this condition.

Some children who suffer from severe JRA may experience long-lasting inflammation that damages the joint surfaces. The result can be the kind of disabling crippling one usually associates with adult *rheumatoid arthritis.*

Prolonged joint inflammation can speed up or slow down the growth of a child's bones, resulting in one bone being longer or shorter than normal. However, growth resumes once the disease has been brought under control.

While inflammation is common to all forms of *juvenile arthritis,* an awareness of the differences between the forms can help you identify and understand the type of arthritis your child may have.

Systemic JRA: About 20 percent of all children with *juvenile rheumatoid arthritis* have this form of the disease. It strikes an equal number of boys and girls and affects children of any age, but especially those under ten. High fevers are a common symptom with the fever usually appearing in the early evening and gradually rising to 103 degrees or higher. After a few hours the temperature comes back down to normal, only to rise again the next evening. Chills and shaking often accompany the fever and your child may indeed feel very sick. Yet sometimes the high fever produces no distress for the child at all. These bouts with fever can last for weeks or even months but rarely persist for more than six months.

A rash may also accompany the fever. This rash can come and go for many days in a row and may appear only when the child's temperature is up or after a bath. The pale red spots of the rash commonly appear on the child's chest and thighs but sometimes show up on other parts of the body as well.

Systemic JRA affects many of the child's joints. These joint problems may begin at the same time as the fever, or they may develop weeks or even months later. Some children report that the pain in their joints increases when they have a fever, and that the pain lessens as the temperature goes down. The joint problems can continue after the period of recurring fever ends and can become a major long-term difficulty for the child if not treated properly.

Other complications of *systemic JRA* include inflammation of the outer lining of the heart; stomach pain; enlargement of the liver, spleen, and lymph glands; anemia; and an excessive number of white blood cells. Regular visits to the doctor are essential to properly monitor and treat these problems. During the acute stage, the child may have to spend long periods in the hospital.

Polyarticular JRA: It's estimated that 40 to 50 percent of all children with *juvenile rheumatoid arthritis* have this form of the disease. Girls get *polyarticular* arthritis more often than boys do. The disease typically begins in five or more joints in the child's fingers and hands, and can also affect the weight-bearing joints such as the hips, knees, ankles, and feet. The affected joints are often symmetrical, meaning that the same joints on both sides of the body are affected simultaneously. Some children experience fevers, but these tend to be far less severe than the high temperatures of *systemic JRA*.

The child with *polyarticular JRA* is also likely to develop lumps on the elbows or any other joint that comes into frequent contact with tables and chairs, or lumps on the feet due to pressure from shoes. This disease is probably identical to adult *rheumatoid arthritis*.

Pauciarticular JRA: Children with the *pauciarticular* variety account for between 30 and 40 percent of all those afflicted with JRA. It begins by affecting only a few joints—four or less—and usually strikes the larger joints, such as the knees, ankles, or elbows. It rarely affects the same joint on both sides of the body. The swollen joints of *pauciarticular JRA* often produce little pain, and the presence of arthritis is frequently detected only by a particularly observant parent.

It is more common in girls and may cause inflammation of the eyes. The symptoms of inflammation—including red eyes, eye pain, and failing vision—don't appear for several months after the inflammation has begun to develop. However, the presence of inflammation can be detected before symptoms develop through an examination done by an eye doctor, or ophthalmologist. If the examination reveals eye inflammation, it can be treated to avoid more serious eye problems.

How Long Does JRA Last?

Juvenile rheumatoid arthritis is considered a "chronic" disease—it can last a long time. Sometimes, JRA never goes away, but, except for the *polyarticular* form, that is highly unusual. It's important for you to realize that the odds are in favor of your child recovering and experiencing no serious or permanent disability. But the process of recovery can take months or even years. In the meantime, you and your whole family must learn to live with the disease. The outlook is optimistic.

In fact, as in some other forms of arthritis, the symptoms of JRA may simply disappear. When this occurs, the disease is said to be in remission, a state that can last years, months, or a lifetime. It doesn't mean the disease itself has gone away, only that the symptoms are dormant. You can't be sure that your child will have a lasting remission, so you must continue to work closely with your doctor.

How Is JRA Diagnosed?

Diagnosis of JRA can be difficult. The symptoms vary from child to child and from one form of the disease to another. Because of this, there are often many steps involved in discovering JRA, and determining what form of the disease is present. The main steps include a review of the medical history, a complete physical examination, laboratory tests, X-rays, and sometimes the examination of joint fluid or tissue.

History. How has your child been feeling? What illness and diseases has he or she had in the past? What are the symptoms of the current illness? Doctors point out that many viruses can cause infections in children which, in turn, can lead to temporary joint problems. In order for a doctor to make an accurate diagnosis, your child must have experienced symptoms for six weeks or more. Your doctor will also want to know if other members of your family have ever had arthritis.

Physical examination. Your family doctor should pay special attention to your child's joints, checking for JRA's telltale signs of inflammation. A child who complains of aches and pains but shows no signs of joint damage probably does not have JRA. The physician should also be looking for other signs, such as the rash that accompanies *systemic JRA,* and the lumps that can appear in *polyarticular JRA*. If there is any suspicion of eye involvement or if *pauciarticular arthritis* is diagnosed, your doctor should refer the child to an eye doctor.

Laboratory tests: Several lab tests can be performed by your doctor, but there is no single test that provides positive proof one way or another.

X-ray examination of joints can be helpful in the course of juvenile arthritis to determine if some other condition—a bone infection, tumor, or fracture—is causing your child's problem. As the disease progresses, the doctor will use X-rays to examine joint damage or changes in bone structure, and, in particular, to track any effect the arthritis might have on bone growth.

A sample of fluid from one or more of your child's joints may be withdrawn with a hollow needle and examined for signs of infection in the joint. On rare occasions, the doctor may perform a biopsy on a joint or lump and analyze the tissue for signs of infection and damage.

As a parent, you may become frustrated because it seems to take so long for the physician to pinpoint your child's ailment. Remember that you can help the diagnostic process by being as specific as possible about your child's problems.

The information you provide makes it easier for the doctor so you may want to keep a notebook record of all your child's symptoms.

Who Should Treat Your Child?

Many parents worry about whether they are taking their child to the doctor who is best qualified to deal with JRA. If he is well-informed about arthritis in children, your family doctor or your regular pediatrician can each do a good job. The doctor who is familiar with your child's medical history, including any previous illnesses or injuries, is usually the best person to see first.

If your child's disease is severe or puzzling, your regular doctor may refer you to a doctor who specializes in arthritis—a rheumatologist—to help with the diagnosis and treatment. Doctors who specialize in JRA are called pediatric rheumatologists. There are fewer than a hundred such doctors in the U.S.

Sometimes it's hard to find a doctor, especially one who specializes in a certain disease. You can ask your county medical society or an accredited hospital in your community to guide you in locating a doctor. Your local chapter of the Arthritis Foundation can help, too.

The American Juvenile Arthritis Organization

In 1981, the Arthritis Foundation set up the American Juvenile Arthritis Organization (AJAO) to focus efforts on the problems related to arthritis in children. The group provides information to the parents and friends of arthritic children as well as health care professionals. Contact your local chapter of the Arthritis Foundation for further information. (See Appendix.)

Ankylosing Spondylitis

This particular variety of arthritis affects your spine. "*Ankylosing*" means stiff or rigid and "*spondyl*" refers to the spine. The spinal inflammation that accompanies this disease can, in the most severe cases, cause the bones of your spine, called *vertebrae,* to fuse or grow together. Fortunately, the majority of cases are mild. Very few people have severe *spondylitis.*

The disease appears to be caused, in part, by inheritance of a particular gene called HLA-B27, which increases the chances of getting *ankylosing spondylitis* two-hundredfold. Since most people who inherit HLA-B27 do not develop the disease, another factor is probably necessary—perhaps a virus infection or a second gene. Its most common symptoms include:

- Constant hip and low back pain, accompanied by stiffness that lasts more than three months.
- If the bones in your neck and hips start to grow together, your ability to do routine chores will become more and more limited.
- Stiffness and soreness in your shoulders, knees, and ankles.
- Fatigue, eye inflammation, and later in the disease, lung and heart problems may develop.
- An exercise program can help you relieve the discomfort caused by *ankylosing spondylitis.* You should consult with your doctor to develop a treatment tailored to your particular ailment.

Scleroderma, the Skin Disease

Scleroderma, also called *progressive systemic sclerosis,* is one of the lesser known diseases associated with arthritis.

The word *scleroderma* literally means "hard skin." It is a disease of the connective tissues which are found in many parts of your body—your skin, blood vessels, joints, and internal organs such as your kidneys, lungs, and bowels.

There are two kinds of *scleroderma:* "localized" or limited, and "systemic" or generalized.

Localized scleroderma affects only limited parts of your body. This condition can usually be found in the skin, muscles, or bones rather than in the internal organs, is relatively mild, and is unlikely to develop into *systemic scleroderma.*

Systemic scleroderma (or *systemic sclerosis*) causes abnormalities in the connective tissues throughout the body. It can occur not only in the skin, but also in the blood vessels, the esophagus (the tube that leads from your mouth to your stomach), stomach, bowels, lungs, kidneys, muscles, and joints. Naturally, with problems in so many major organs, serious complications can occur.

Scleroderma differs from person to person. A patient who has the systemic form may have one or more body parts affected to different degrees. It is difficult for doctors to predict how the disease will develop in each individual.

What Are the Causes?

The direct cause is unknown. Doctors do know that it is not inherited or passed on from one generation to another, except in very rare instances.

It is known that the connective tissues of *scleroderma* sufferers produce excessive amounts of a protein called *collagen.* Think of *collagen* as the woven threads that make up the cloth of a tissue. In *scleroderma,* excess *collagen* is deposited in the skin and in the body organs. And these deposits cause thickening and hardening of the skin.

Scientists believe that the body's immune system plays a part in causing *collagen* deposits. The immune system, as we discussed earlier, is your body's natural defense against disease, and creates antibodies in your blood to fight off bacteria and viruses. But in some people, the immune system attacks and damages cells. Antibodies to some body constituents have been found in people with *scleroderma,* but scientists do not know if they cause the disease in any way. A third feature of *scleroderma* is a narrowing of the small blood vessels throughout the body. The loss of blood supply that results may be responsible for the buildup of *collagen* in connective tissue. The blood vessel narrowing does lead to a marked susceptibility to cold temperatures.

Who Has Scleroderma?

About 100,000 people in the U.S. have *scleroderma.* Women are affected two to three times more often than men. It usually strikes during the prime of life, between the ages of twenty and forty, and is only occasionally seen in children and the elderly.

What Are the Symptoms?

An early symptom of *scleroderma* is *Raynaud's phenomenon,* named after the man who first discovered it. It is an extreme sensitivity to cold, and is most obvious in the fingers. About 90 percent of people with *scleroderma* have this symptom at one time or another. In *Raynaud's phenomenon,* the blood vessels narrow in response to cold or to emotional upset. Sometimes all it takes to trigger this reaction is for the person to walk into a cold room or reach into a refrigerator.

The narrowing of the blood vessels greatly reduces the blood supply to the fingers, causing them to turn very pale. Tingling, numbness, or a cold sensation is felt in the fingers. When the hands warm up, the blood vessels open and skin color becomes blue and then slowly returns to normal as the blood supply to the fingers improves.

Another common symptom of *scleroderma* is swelling or puffiness in the hands and feet, especially in the morning. The skin of your fingers and toes may look and feel swollen. Your normal skin wrinkles may disappear and the skin itself may appear shiny.

About 95 percent of people with *scleroderma* have some kind of thickening and hardening of the skin, especially in the hands, arms, and face. Ulcers on the fingers, a result of the reduced blood supply, sometimes occur. Some people will also develop small, white calcium deposits on the bones of their fingers.

Scleroderma can also cause joint inflammation and pain, stiffness, swelling, warmth, and tenderness. Muscle weakness can also be a sign of *scleroderma.* As the disease progresses, the joints in your hands and other parts of your body usually tighten into a bent position.

This tightening is caused by the hardening of the skin and *also* involves the tissues surrounding the joint.

In rare instances, a person with *scleroderma* may not have any of these obvious symptoms. The disease may only affect the connective tissues of the digestive system, or some other internal body system, leaving the skin and joints untouched. When *scleroderma* strikes the digestive system, the muscles in your esophagus may become weak, making it difficult to swallow and pass food down to the stomach. Heartburn can be a frequent problem, causing a burning feeling in the back of the throat and esophagus.

The condition may also affect the bowels and lungs. High blood pressure is yet another indicator and may occur if the kidneys are damaged.

Obviously, *scleroderma* can involve a complex tangle of problems. The only way to treat the disease is through careful consultation with your doctor.

How Does a Doctor Diagnose Scleroderma?

As with any attempt at diagnosis, the first step is a thorough physical examination and a study of past and present symptoms.

Laboratory and other tests will be needed to help to determine if you have *scleroderma,* and whether it is present in your internal organs. No single test will prove the presence of *scleroderma.* One of the tests a doctor may perform is a *biopsy,* the removal of a small piece of skin to examine it under a microscope for signs of *scleroderma.* The doctor will also probably X-ray and perhaps check the muscle pressure of your esophagus to detect if your digestive system is involved.

Studies of lung or heart function are also performed frequently.

Systemic Lupus Erythematosus

Systemic lupus erythematosus is a disease that affects an estimated 100,000 Americans, 90 percent of them women, according to the Arthritis Foundation. If uncontrolled, it can damage the skin, joints, and internal organs. Usually called simply *lupus,* it can lead to serious problems if it is not diagnosed and treated early.

At the onset of *lupus,* its symptoms may come and go with no definite pattern. Fever, weakness, weight loss, and fatigue may be its first warning signs. A rash often appears on the face, neck, or arms. Other early signs may also include joint pains, muscle aches, swollen glands, lack of appetite, nausea, and vomiting. Some people with *lupus* become extremely sensitive to sunlight, which may make rashes appear or cause existing rashes to worsen. Other factors that may trigger *lupus* flare-ups include minor infections, certain drugs—especially hydralazine for high blood pressure and procainamide for heart disease—emotional upsets, and pregnancy.

As *lupus* develops, some people develop inflammation of the linings of body organs, especially of the lungs, heart, and abdomen. Uncontrolled, *lupus* can also cause damage to the kidneys, nerves and the brain.

Because *lupus* can cause so many complications, early diagnosis and continuing medical treatment is essential.

"Dallas" Star's Mother Tormented by Crippling Disease

Victoria (Pamela Ewing) Principal lives in the shadow of a frightening disease—lupus. She says she is already showing symptoms of the sometimes devastating illness, which has plagued her mother for years. Victoria, who is national campaign chairperson for the Arthritis Foundation, tells of her mother's brave battle against lupus in her own words.

"I've wept over the suffering my mother has undergone in her battle against the disease. The weakness, the blinding headaches, the days and weeks flat on her back, the terrible rashes from being in sunlight.

"And I know the very same illness may strike me—doctors say the tendency to have lupus may be hereditary. Already I have some symptoms of lupus, but I pray I won't have it as bad as my mom does, and I don't think I will. She was nineteen when it started. Doctors didn't know much about it then. There was no name for what my mother had. But she very wisely listened to her own body, and realized, long before the doctors did, she had to take extra good care of herself.

"I remember as a child, I couldn't understand what was happening to her. One day she'd seem so vital and healthy, we'd go outside and play baseball. Then suddenly, my mother would be in bed for two weeks. I didn't know this was a symptom of the disease."

At its worst, Victoria said, lupus kept her mother ill, flat on her back, up to twenty-eight days a month. But ten years ago her mom began to limit the amount of time she spent outdoors during the day, to avoid exposure to sunlight. She began to rest and exercise regularly. The results were dramatic.

"Today she's ill about eight days out of the month," Victoria said. "But she's not a hermit. We occasionally go out during the day. She wears dark glasses, a sunblock on her skin and carries an umbrella.

"She suffers, but she's fighting it. She's a strong, courageous woman. She's not dying from lupus, but it is still life-endangering. She faces the fear that the disease could spread to other organs. And as I look at her, I have to realize that I could also wind up suffering like her."

To stay as healthy as possible, Victoria has had to put the brakes on her once-frenzied way of life. "I've had to adjust to a different life-style," she said. "I used to squeeze as much activity as I could into the time I had. But now I've learned to rest, to slow down. I've learned to give my body a rest—to give it a chance to fight off the onset of the disease that struck my mother.

"Sure, fear of lupus might be ticking away in me like a mental time bomb, but I don't dwell on it. I have to take a positive attitude. I do everything I can to take care of myself. Focusing my whole life on what might happen would only deplete my energy. Besides, Arthritis Foundation researchers are learning more about lupus and how to control it all the time. Rest, exercise, and special drugs can help. The advice of a physician who's an expert on lupus—like the one I go to—is essential.

"I've tried to incorporate my work for the Foundation into everything I do outside of 'Dallas.' Arthritis isn't limited to the old. I want the world to know how painful and debilitating arthritis can be, and how it can strike anyone, even someone like me!"

Psoriatic Arthritis

Psoriatic arthritis is a form of arthritis that can accompany the skin condition called *psoriasis,* which causes red patches and rashes on the body. About 5 percent of people with *psoriasis* will also develop arthritis. For most people the symptoms of arthritis are mild and require little treatment. For a few people, however, the disease can become severe. *Psoriatic arthritis* is particularly likely to affect the fingers or the spine. In the spine, it is very similar to *ankylosing spondylitis.*

Treatment can include rest, exercise, and drugs for the skin and the arthritis pain and inflammation. Surgery to repair or replace the damaged joints is seldom done.

Infectious Arthritis

Just as *psoriatic arthritis* can follow the skin disorder *psoriasis, infectious arthritis* can follow other diseases such as viral, bacterial, and fungal infections. *Infectious arthritis* is a complication of another disease. The develops is that an infectious agent first cause disease and then spreads into one or more joints, causing arthritis.

For example, one common cause of adult *infectious arthritis* is the bacterium that causes gonorrhea. In some people, this bacterium escapes from the genital organs and gets into the bloodstream. Through the blood it is carried to the joints and leads to arthritis.

Drug treatment to get rid of the infection usually clears up the arthritis completely, if treatment is begun soon after the joint symptoms begin. If the infection in a joint is not treated right away, however, the joint may become badly damaged.

Fibrositis, Tendonitis, and Bursitis

As we mentioned at the start of this chapter, these three disorders are included in the larger category called rheumatic diseases. *Fibrositis, tendonitis,* and *bursitis* affect the supportive tissues around the joint, not the joint itself.

Fibrositis is a very common condition that may not really deserve to be called a disease. The word refers to pain in the muscles, ligaments, and tendons that has no apparent cause. While there is pain, and the functioning of the joint can be affected by the pain, there are no signs of damage to the joint in *fibrositis.* In the U.S., more than seven million people—more women than men—are affected by the disorder. It usually strikes between the ages of thirty-five and sixty. Most frequently *fibrositis* goes away by itself, but it can last anywhere from weeks or months, to years. The pain in this disorder results from the tightening of the muscles in one or more areas. Treatment can include physical therapy, exercise, and drugs to reduce the pain, help you to sleep, and fight depression.

Bursitis and *tendonitis* are painful conditions that usually last only a short time without causing permanent damage. *Bursitis* means inflammation of a bursa (the small sac which acts like a cushion between muscles, and between muscle and bone), and *tendonitis* means inflammation of the tendons. Both conditions often start suddenly. Almost all episodes stop within a matter of days or weeks. If treated correctly, there is seldom any lasting damage. Some people seem to have repeated attacks of *tendonitis* and *bursitis* which can occur in the same part of the body or in another, previously unaffected part. There are an estimated two to three million people who get these conditions each year, although the actual figure could be much higher. Long-term joint stress and normal wear and tear in the process of aging are often cited as possible causes of *tendonitis* and *bursitis.*

Both disorders can occur singly or together. The main symptom for each is pain, although in severe cases swelling may also occur. Treatment usually includes rest, hot and cold treatments, medication to reduce pain and inflammation, and exercise. Although the shoulder is the most commonly affected area in *bursitis* and *tendonitis,* the well-known "tennis elbow" and "housemaid's knee" are common forms of *tendonitis* and *bursitis,* respectively.

Polymyalgia Rheumatica (PMR), Polymyositis, and Dermatomyositis

These three diseases all affect the muscles. *Polymyalgia Rheumatica* (PMR) causes certain groups of muscles to be stiff and painful. *Poly* means *many, myo* means *muscle, algia* means *pain,* and *rheumatica* refers to inflammation of the connective tissues such as muscles and bones. Though PMR is chronic and there is no cure for this disease, it may eventually go away for no apparent reason. Most often, the illness lasts for two years, although it can be present for a time period of a few months to many years. The disorder, which occurs almost always in people over fifty, starts with flu-like symptoms—aching, stiff muscles and joints, especially in the shoulders, hip, and neck areas. PMR often occurs together with a disease called *Giant Cell Arteritis,* which causes inflammation and narrowing of some of the arteries in the body, particularly in the scalp and the head. Since *Giant Cell Arteritis* can cause blindness if not treated in time, it is important to be sure that a person with PMR does not have this additional disease. A biopsy of an artery in the scalp may be needed to determine whether this complication is present.

The cause of PMR is not known, though some scientists believe heredity may play a part. The most effective drugs for treating PMR are the corticosteroids, which are similar to the hormones your body produces naturally. Most people will receive the steroid drug called prednisone, often in large doses at first.

Frequently this treatment results in rapid improvement within a few days. Once improvement is shown the dosage will be gradually reduced. For those who don't need corticosteroids, aspirin can relieve the pain and reduce swelling. Exercise and rest are also part of the treatment program.

In *polymyositis* the main problems are weakness and inflammation of the muscles. These are the same major problems in *dermatomyositis* which also includes a skin *(derma)* rash. The term *myositis* refers to both of these illnesses. *Myositis* is chronic, but with proper treatment and management it can be brought under control. Both illnesses result in damage to some of the body's connective tissue, mainly in the muscles, and the major result is weakness. The causes of both *polymyositis* and *dermatomyositis* are not known, but some scientists think the immune system and viral infection may be involved. These diseases are not very common. In the U.S., it is thought that five people out of every one million get some form of *myositis*. Twice as many women are affected as men, and although people of any age can get these disorders, most adults with *myositis* are between thirty and sixty, and most children with it are between five and fifteen.

Myositis begins and progresses in many different ways, but for the majority the problems come on slowly over a period of several years. The symptoms often come and go for no apparent reason. The muscles most likely to be involved are in the hip and shoulder areas. A person with *dermatomyositis* may develop a patchy, reddish rash on the face, around the eyes, on the knuckles and elbows, and sometimes on the knees and ankles. Some people also have puffy eyelids as a result of this illness. Other symptoms of *myositis* may be fever, weight loss, and some pain and tenderness in muscles and joints. *Myositis* is difficult to diagnose because it resembles several other muscle diseases. The treatment process includes corticosteroids, physical therapy, exercise, and rest.

CHAPTER X

Arthritis Research

IN EARLIER CHAPTERS WE OUTLINED THE BEST-known and time-tested therapies using drugs, surgery, and exercise. These therapies are the result of years of research and experimentation in the scientific, medical, and business communities across America and around the world. Now let's take a look at where we stand in the battle against arthritis, what we know, what we don't know, and what directions scientists are headed in, in their search for the answers.

Research on a great scientific puzzle like arthritis falls into three stages.

- *The first stage* is description. Scientists try to find and list all the things that are actually present in the trouble spot. In arthritis, the scientists list all the things that are present in a diseased joint, but are not found in a normal joint.
- *In the second stage,* an attempt is made to fit the pieces of the puzzle together, to relate them to each other and put them into a logical structure and sequence of events that will reveal how disease developed in the joint.

• *In the third stage,* the correctness of the proposed structure and sequence of events is tested under controlled conditions.

Research into *rheumatoid arthritis*—to take just one example—is at stage three; that's where the big answers are. Stage three research focuses on the process of inflammation, which, like all life processes, is incredibly complex.

To understand just how complex inflammation is, try to imagine having to make a map of every avenue, street, and alley in a major metropolitan city, and of every highway leading into and out of it; learn all the patterns of traffic flow; determine the starting point and destination of every car, truck, and bus traveling these roads; discover the reason for each roadblock that causes traffic snarls and detours; and determine the detour routes taken and the consequences of delay for each vehicle.

Only with knowledge of how the whole bewildering system works, under normal and abnormal conditions, could one even begin to pinpoint the alternate routes and flow of traffic that lead to the process of disease.

Although inflammation in *rheumatoid arthritis* has patterns unique to that particular disease, inflammation in the broad sense is a process common to many human disorders. Inflammation appears every time the body reacts to an injury, and there are countless diseases besides *rheumatoid arthritis* in which inflammation is present. Solving all the mysteries of inflammation would be one of the greatest achievements of the twentieth century.

As arthritis research progresses in its third and final

stage, scientists are moving toward unlocking two great secrets.

- First, as we've discussed before, what is the mysterious "thing" that causes the *rheumatoid arthritis* process to start? It is often referred to as the "unknown trigger," and some suspect it is a virus. Identifying it, and finding a way to fight it, is one path to the ultimate goal—a prevention or cure for *rheumatoid arthritis.*
- Second, there may be another path to finding a cure, and many scientists think that a breakthrough will come in this area more quickly than in the search to identify and neutralize the "trigger," or the path described above.

The question is: Can a safe drug be devised to break the chain reaction process of inflammation at key points, thus bringing it to a halt and preventing joint damage?

This theoretical drug would provide a treatment that would work even if research had not yet revealed the "trigger" that starts the process of inflammation. The more scientists learn about inflammation, the more hopeful and realistic the possibility of a completely effective drug becomes.

The Experimental Process

Experiments are a critical aspect of research, and they are done for a number of reasons. They are a means of demonstrating something which is known to be true. They are a way to determine whether something—such as a theory—is true or valid. And they are used to determine whether something new can produce certain desired results. Complicated, isn't it? In simpler terms an experiment is a kind of test. Research involves experiments to test the value and effectiveness of new drugs, surgical procedures, and other methods of treatment. These experiments are designed to test not only the good effects but the bad effects as well. It is only after years of experiments involving hundreds of thousands of people that a decision can be made about whether the solution—the theory, the drug, the surgical technique—solves a problem, or solves a problem but creates too many or too severe new problems to be useful, or is ultimately worthless.

A major complicating factor in the process of experimentation is that there is often a bewildering array of contradictory results. Take aspirin for instance. For some people aspirin is the best drug for treating the symptoms of arthritis. For others, as we have seen, aspirin not only doesn't effectively alleviate the symptoms, it can create adverse reactions or side effects. In this instance, the contradictory results did not mean aspirin was not a valuable and successful form of treatment, it simply meant that aspirin would not be the drug of choice for some people.

The reason for this contradiction is clear: Each and every one of us is different. That means not only do we have the obvious differences in appearance, for example, but we also demonstrate our dissimilarities in how we react to drugs or other therapies.

The experimental process involves evaluating these contradictions: Are they important, incidental, prevalent, isolated, and so forth? Clearly, in the case of aspirin, they were judged to be important enough to warn people about, but not prevalent enough to warrant abandoning the use of the drug. Other times, the contradictions can be more baffling. For instance, a new treatment tried on a research group in Los Angeles will seem to be successful, while the same treatment will fail miserably with a group in Detroit. Why? It could be the way the study or experiment was conducted, the quality of the product being tested, the supervision of the scientists, the background of the people testing the treatment, the place where the experiment took place, the follow-up and questions asked, and a thousand other variables. One of the best ways to narrow down the possibilities is to continue repeating the experiment and narrowing down the causes and significance of the contradictions.

Clearly, it is only after years of checking and rechecking the results of experiments that a form of therapy or a treatment is finally judged favorably and made available to the general public. There are reasons for all this careful work, and the primary reason is your safety.

Standards have been set up to insure the public's safety. The ones we are most familiar with are fire protection standards, health codes, sanitary regulations, and building codes, just to name a few. They may give us a pain in the neck, but they do save countless lives every day. In scientific research there are safety measures as well. These standards must be met before an experimental treatment is judged to be a safe and effective treatment, and an acceptable form of therapy for the general public.

One of the standards imposed on scientists is the *double-blind trial*. In a standard experiment for a new pain-relieving drug, there would be a researcher administering the drug, and a group of people taking the drug. The role of the researcher would then be to note any effects the drug had on each person. There might be a reduction in pain, an increase in pain, an unrelated reaction such as the development of a headache, or no reaction at all. In a *double-blind trial* neither the researcher nor the people in the experiment would know when or if the actual drug was being administered. The researcher is given three pills at three different periods of the day, for example. They all look alike, yet one is made from sugar, one from a vitamin, and one is the new drug X. Since they all look alike, no one in the experiment knows which is which. Only the person giving the pills to the researcher would know. It may sound silly at first, but think about it for a minute.

With both the conductor of the experiment *and* the subjects "blind" to the identity of the real drug, any prejudice or bias in favor of the drug is ruled out, and the results of the experiment are "pure," or untainted. What if the researcher does know he is giving drug X? Maybe he is excited about this new drug and his eyes seem to get bigger when he is administering it, or maybe he smiles a little—all unknown to him and involuntarily. The subjects in the experiment could pick up on this smile or wide-eyed hint—even subconsciously. Then the results would be biased, and the experiment worthless.

One of the influences at work may be the *placebo effect.* Simply put, this is the power of the mind over the body. The subject knows—as a result of the researcher's expression—that he is taking drug X. He wants drug X to work and as a result he believes it does work.

It has been proved over and over that people who want to get better, and who believe that a new remedy can help, often do get better—temporarily. Scientific studies show that people often experience improvement in their condition after injesting a harmless and ineffective substance simply because they believe they are getting real medicine. This psychological effect is only temporary. Because of the presence of the *placebo effect* in the above example the findings of the experiment are prejudiced in favor of drug X. *Double-blind trials* can save experiments from such prejudices and many more. These trials ensure the integrity, or soundness, of such experiments and are a crucial standard that has to be met before any treatment is approved by the medical profession.

Experimental Treatments

It is important that you keep in mind the uncertainty of experimental treatments. They are part of the trial and error process which leads to both failure and success. It is the hope of success in solving some of the mysteries of disease that drives scientists, doctors, researchers, government agencies, and the private sector to develop experimental treatments and to test them out. Some of the early findings can generate a lot of excitement privately and publicly. The media and the public have a tremendous thirst for discoveries and hopeful cures, and as a result the world of science is both an exotic and potent force in all our lives. When we are sick, incapacitated, or have a chronic illness, the desire for quick fixes and sudden turnarounds can overpower our common sense. Too often we neglect what we *know* in favor of what we *hope* is so.

For the rest of this chapter, we will review some of the many recent areas of research in arthritis. Just remember that these are experimental treatments. You may wish to discuss some of these ideas with your doctor, but NONE OF THE EXPERIMENTAL TREATMENTS DISCUSSED BELOW SHOULD BE USED OR IMITATED WITHOUT THE ADVICE AND CONSENT OF YOUR DOCTOR.

Experimental Drug Therapies

New drugs are being developed continuously to treat the symptoms of arthritis. Though many are not yet approved for therapeutic use, and cannot be obtained except to conduct clinical research, they may provide hope in the future for arthritis treatment. Other drugs have been put through rigorous testing and are awaiting approval from the Food and Drug Administration. They are not available for widespread distribution legally and cannot be used, except under care by a doctor participating in the tests.

New painkilling chemicals that may prove to help in the fight against arthritic pain are: *Buturphanol tartate,* available as an injection, and purported to be non-addictive, seems to have fewer of the side effects, such as drowsiness, that other painkillers have; *D-Phenylalanine* (DLPA), said to be a painkiller effective in treating *osteoarthritis* and *rheumatoid arthritis; Orgotein,* a drug which is said to reduce swelling and stiffness as well as pain, when injected directly into the diseased joint.

Three drugs called *Cytoxan, Imuran,* and *Plaquenil*

are combined in a new experimental treatment to halt the spread of joint damage in patients with severe *rheumatoid arthritis.* Only a small number of patients have thus far been treated with this combination.

Another potential therapy involves giving cortisone-like drugs. MPPT—which stands for (the drug) *Methylprednisolone* pulse therapy—involves administering a large single dose of the drug intravenously (pulse) at regular intervals. One UCLA doctor cites "dramatic" results in reducing inflammation. Although methylprednisolene has long been known to be effective in reducing the inflammation of *rheumatoid arthritis,* this treatment cannot be evaluated until the long-term side effects are known.

A new gold-containing drug called *Auranofin* does not have to be injected into the muscle but can be taken orally. It appears to produce fewer side effects than injectable gold and also to be about as effective.

Antibiotics

An antibiotic used worldwide to fight tuberculosis may provide some relief when injected into the knees of people with *rheumatoid arthritis.* Currently, injections of steroids are often used to treat severe knee inflammation. But research by Dr. Innocenso Caruso of Italy suggests that a limited series of injections of the tuberculosis drug *rifamycin SV* eliminates *rheumatoid knee synovitis* indefinitely—without need of further treatments.

For this drug to be used for arthritis treatment in the United States it would have to go through testing in American hospitals and be approved by the Food and

Drug Administration. If it is approved by the FDA, it could be available in the next few years.

Radiation Therapy

Rheumatoid arthritis sufferers whose ailment has defied all other treatments may be offered new hope with a still-developing radiation treatment that has been experimented with at Stanford and Harvard universities.

Some people who've undergone the radiation have actually started walking after being dependent on wheelchairs or crutches.

The treatment, according to Stanford scientists, consists of a brief exposure to radiation daily over the course of five or six weeks.

Dr. Samuel Strober, associate professor of medicine at Stanford, reported that, "At least two men and one woman who came to us were unable to walk without assistance. Within several months after the treatment, these three were able to walk well enough so that they didn't need crutches."

The radiation focuses on the body's immune system which is known to play a role in *rheumatoid arthritis.* Larger studies involving more patients are being set up, as well as studies comparing people who receive the treatment with similar people who are on standard forms of treatment.

Electric Current

A box the size of a cigarette pack that emits electrical pulses has been found in one study to be effective in relieving pain in people with *rheumatoid arthritis.* The study was conducted by Dr. V. Nanda Kumar, of the Veterans Administration Medical Center in Kansas City, Missouri. In a process called TENS (transcutaneous electrical nerve stimulation), the box emits twelve to one hundred pulses of electricity per second through two electrodes attached to the inflamed joint to stimulate the nerves.

In the study done by Dr. Kumar, who is clinical associate professor of physical medicine and rehabilitation at the University of Kansas, and Dr. John W. B. Redford, a professor in the same field at the University, twenty people with *rheumatoid arthritis* were asked to lift a weight before and after their TENS treatment in their wrists. The results: 80 percent or sixteen wrists showed "definite improvement" in the ability to lift the weight and to hold it. Eight of the wrists doubled in strength and another four improved by 50 percent.

Hypnosis

When other forms of treatment have failed, hypnosis has been used successfully to help temporarily relieve the aches and pains associated with arthritis. By being hypnotized, or by hypnotizing themselves, people can calm themselves down, relieve tension and stress, and often block out the pain for a few hours.

Blood Filtering (Apheresis)

Some medical researchers have reported that they can reduce the inflammation in some people with *rheumatoid arthritis* by using an unusual technique: filtering the person's own blood. The technique, called *apheresis,* involves pumping one's blood through a machine that separates out different components such as lymphocytes and plasma. Then the rest of the blood is pumped back into the same person's body.

Doctors at the National Institutes of Health say they aren't sure how this process helps pain and stiffness, or if it does. But they think that some white blood cells, or lymphocytes, are part of what causes the problem in inflamed joints. Perhaps by removing these cells temporarily (the body manufactures new ones quickly to replace the ones taken out), a person's condition can improve.

A few people who have undergone the blood filtering treatment reported immediate relief, and in some the relief lasted quite awhile. However, in three studies in which people were divided into two groups, one receiving *apheresis* and the other a sham (fake) *apheresis,* there was no difference in the benefit seen in the two groups.

Ant Venom

The venom of Bolivia's Devil Tree ants—once used to torture natives to death—is being tested by medical researchers at the University of Miami as a weapon against the pain of *rheumatoid arthritis.*

The mysterious treatment was first tested on thirty people in the Dominican Republic several years ago, and twenty-three of the thirty improved. The researchers there reported that a few people had astonishingly good results.

One man, about forty, had classic *rheumatoid arthritis.* He had been a cowboy, but his disease had rendered him immobile. After taking the venom, the man was back at his job and on his horse in a matter of weeks. In another baffling case, a horribly deformed woman showed dramatic improvement after being injected with the venom.

It all began, apparently, when a German doctor who lived in the area noticed that Bolivians allowed themselves to suffer a few bites from the tiny ants to cure their aches and pains. The doctor brought the phenomenon to the attention of researchers.

Preliminary studies at the University of Miami are promising, but the eventual value of this treatment is unknown. If it works it may be difficult to extract and purify enough venom to be of any practical use.

Acupuncture

The Arthritis Foundation warns that acupuncture is a waste of time and money, but some people claim to have found relief through this ancient Chinese practice of placing needles into the body at strategic points, and there has been some research done in this area.

According to three different studies conducted by the Arthritis Foundation, "Acupuncture does not work on the disease process of arthritis at all, and the only benefit scientists found was the 'placebo effect.'"

Cold Therapy

In an unorthodox approach to treating *rheumatoid arthritis,* a Japanese doctor says that he has achieved remarkable success with the use of freezing cold and exercise. Patients spend two to three minutes once or twice a day in a minus 228-degree Fahrenheit chamber while exercising vigorously.

Laser Therapy

It has been reported that Soviet doctors are using laser beams to help relieve suffering in arthritis patients.

Dr. Viktor Inyushin, of Russia's Scientific Research Center of Biophysics, reported that the revolutionary technique is a combination of space-age laser technology and acupuncture.

"A laser beam is directed both at the affected joints and at certain acupuncture points for periods of five to fifteen seconds," said Dr. Inyushin. "Meanwhile, the patient feels absolutely nothing." Some American scientists are interested in the Soviet discovery.

After successive treatments over a period of many months, the Soviets reported that their patients had improved considerably. Over 90 percent of the people returned to their homes completely rehabilitated, they said. (However, no control studies were done to confirm these findings.)

CHAPTER XI

Quackery in Arthritis

QUACKERY CAN BE A DANGEROUS AND DEADLY game. Most often you are simply robbed of your money and your self-esteem. But sometimes you can be robbed of your health or even your life.

Maybe that simple, straightforward sentence can save you from making a big mistake. No matter what you read, what you hear, dream, think, imagine, or want to believe—the facts can't be changed. If and when they are, you can't possibly miss them. The medical establishment will celebrate it, the federal government will verify it, the drug companies will fill our eyes and ears with news of it.

Until then, every time you hear of a "cure-all" a "special, mysterious, miraculous, exclusive" treatment that will make you whole again without a trace of disease, disfigurement, soreness, stiffness, inflammation, or any other damage—grab your pocket book and run! This is no laughing matter.

Quackery is a form of theft. It will rob you of hope,

faith, peace of mind, your pay check and maybe even your life. And there's really no way to stop it. As long as there is one person left on earth who believes that a miracle cure can come in a tub full of kerosene or a tube of horse liniment, quackery will thrive.

And quackery isn't just the result of foolishness. Sure we are all silly sometimes and take a chance on something that's pretty ridiculous. But quackery in medicine feeds not on the foolish, but on the desperate. It's one thing to buy an oil potion to make your fingernails grow two inches long in one week, and quite another to spend your savings on injections of illegal drugs. Failure in the first instance has the impact of a practical joke. Failure in the second is dangerous.

If you have arthritis and your treatment is not effective in relieving the symptoms, you can become frantic. Pain can make the strongest men cry, and the bravest cower in fear. But what ought to make you even more frantic is the thought that people are out there trying to profit from your suffering and misery. They don't care if you get better. Quacks couldn't care less what happens to you—they just want your money. And they get it:

- Quackery and unproven remedy sales cost arthritis sufferers one *billion* dollars each year.
- For every dollar spent on legitimate research this year, twenty-five dollars will go to unfounded arthritis remedies.
- Quack treatments for arthritis are more numerous than for any other disease.

What Is Quackery?

When a "remedy" is touted as something that it isn't, that's quackery. A copper bracelet is only jewelry until someone claims that it is a cure for arthritis. Because that claim has little, if any, basis in fact and there is absolutely no certifiable proof, it is quackery.

In days gone by, quacks selling potions and tonics from town to town were easy to identify by their fast sales pitches and gaudy wagons. Today, the typical quack speaks a more sophisticated language of medical technology and can often appear legitimate.

Claims made by quacks can be surprisingly subtle and shrewd. Very often, there is someone who claims to be a medical spokesman in the forefront—what the Arthritis Foundation calls a "white coat connection"—who makes the quackery seem legitimate.

Of course, there is also a lot of old-fashioned quackery going on like the arthritis "cure" advertisements you sometimes see. In addition, there is also misleading and sensationalized publicity for drugs that are legitimate but haven't been fully tested yet. This sensationalism can raise false hopes—about how soon the drug will be available, for example—just as much as outright quackery can. And there are hundreds of remedies of every description that some people claim have been effective, but have no medical basis on which to substantiate this claim.

It can sometimes be difficult to identify quack remedies. While some are obviously foolish, others have some degree of medical backing. For example, although copper bracelets can't cure arthritis, there is scientific evidence that certain metals have an effect on arthritis. The fact remains, however, that you're not going to absorb enough metal through your skin to do any good—if you could easily absorb copper by wearing it, its side effects would probably make you very ill.

As far as safety is concerned, quack remedies can range from harmless to near-lethal—and a few are so toxic they can lead to death.

How can you tell the difference between true and false claims? Between the harmless and lethal? There are certain things to watch out for. Be suspicious of extraordinary claims of cures by simply using:

- *Vaccines.* There's no such thing as a vaccine for arthritis.
- *Hormones.* Both male and female hormones are very powerful and potentially dangerous drugs. They should be prescribed only by your doctor, if they're to be used at all.
- *Fad diets and food supplements.* Nutritionally sound food can make you feel better generally. But "Miracle Cures" attributed to diets and herbs and vitamins are highly suspicious. Research is going on around the world to establish just what benefits, if any, can be attributed to diets and natural food supplements.
- *Medical "discoveries."* Drugs like *Liefcort* and *Gerovital H3* may be great discoveries for the bank accounts of entrepreneurs, but they can be extremely harmful to arthritic.

• *Ointments.* Rubs, lotions, liniments, and other locally applied remedies may help alleviate a little pain and tenderness, but they aren't cures in themselves.

• *Devices.* Although some devices can help people with arthritis avoid joint stress, no device can serve as a cure.

• *Sea products.* Seawater, mussel extracts, and seaweed bracelets have been promoted as arthritis cures. They simply aren't.

• *Mail-order cures.* Be suspicious of anyone who advertises and sells medicines, potions, and "cures" through the mail. If the product is legitimate, why isn't it at the local drug store?

What's the Harm in Trying the Offbeat?

The danger involved in "offbeat" remedies depends on the treatment itself. Many remedies are quite harmless and inexpensive, especially those based on folklore remedies or recipes passed on down through generations of a family. Other treatments, especially those involving drugs, can be very dangerous. And all quack remedies, regardless of risks, cost money that could have been put to far better use.

Every time you substitute a quack remedy for a proven treatment, you're postponing the day when you will get proper arthritis treatment. And every day counts in terms of damage and suffering. By spending your time and energy pursuing quack treatments, you may be allowing your disease to get progressively worse, and deformities may progress past the point where they can be corrected.

Tips on How to Spot a Phony

Before you try any new arthritis treatment, be cautious, even suspicious, and check it out. There are many people with various degrees, including some doctors, who profess to have solutions to arthritis. Even if a doctor's credentials make the claim seem legitimate, you should still be alert for the following warning signs of quackery:

1. *A cure for all forms of arthritis is claimed.* Since each form is different and has a different cause, no one treatment could work for all forms.

2. *The cure or remedy is described as a "secret" formula or device,* or the words "exclusive" and "special" are used. Honest scientists don't keep their discoveries secret or exclusive.

3. *Only testimonials or personal case histories are cited* from people who claim the remedy is effective. When these histories are offered as sole proof of the effectiveness of the remedy, beware. Testimonials are opinion, not proof.

4. *Quick, simple relief of pain is promised or implied.* There's nothing simple or quick about controlling the pain of arthritis.

5. *The treatment is promoted as "cleansing" the body* of poisons or toxins, allowing the body's natural curative powers to clear up arthritis.

6. *Drugs and/or surgery are condemned* as damaging, dangerous, and unnecessary, and the patient is advised to try a nondrug program. That's just playing on your fears of drugs and surgery.

7. *No reliable evidence or scientific proof is offered* to back up claims that the remedy is safe and effective. This indicates that the promoter has not had the method properly tested in clinical trials.

8. *A special diet or nutrition program is promoted as the cure* for arthritis. Except in the case of *gout,* research scientists have not found that any foods or nutrients can aggravate or relieve arthritis alone.

9. *The "medical establishment" is accused of conspiracy* to thwart progress by refusing to recognize or approve the remedy being promoted. Particular targets include the Arthritis Foundation, the American Medical Association, and the Food and Drug Administration, all quite legitimate organizations devoted to responsible health care.

Media Promotion

Not so long ago, word of "revolutionary" arthritis remedies traveled by word of mouth, from person to person. Although that still happens sometimes, many of today's questionable arthritis treatments appear in the media, as the subject of news and specific ads. People often hear about a "new" arthritis drug or therapy on television, or see it reported in newspapers and magazines.

Newspapers and TV often bring us the preliminary reports on medical treatments before the final verdict is in. The promise of a new and exciting drug makes exciting news, but it also brings with it the powerful, subconscious message that it is a "legitimate" drug. We remember it vaguely until one day we see an ad selling it or drug or remedy that sounds like it, and we are hooked.

But you don't have to make this mistake. Educate yourself about arthritis and you'll be better able to distinguish between the treatments that can help you and those that may harm you.

Testimonial statements praising unproven arthritis remedies can sound very convincing but shouldn't be regarded as "proof" that a remedy works. Here's why:

- No two people are exactly alike in the way they react to any medication or therapy.
- You can't tell if people were taking some other medication at the time which made them feel better, rather than the "cure" that is being given credit.
- Arthritis has flare-ups and remissions and often appears to go away by itself. A remission may occur spontaneously just as someone tries a new treatment, leading him to believe that the treatment has worked.
- As many as 50 percent of arthritis sufferers get better no matter what they take, thanks to the power of the mind over the body, or the placebo effect.

Historic Quack Devices

There have been so many wacky devices purporting to cure diseases that a National Museum of Medical Quackery has been established in St. Louis, Missouri. Among the items on display at the museum are:

- *The Orgone Energy Accumulator*—Named by the FDA as "One of the greatest medical frauds of all time." It's a coffin-sized box designed by behavioral psychologist Wilhelm Reich.

"Orgone simply doesn't exist," said Dr. Brodeur, spokesman for the museum. "But Reich claimed that it was a cosmic force that made people healthy. His theory was that if a person wasn't feeling well he had lost some of his orgone and had to be recharged." By simply sitting in the box, even cancer victims could be cured, Reich claimed.

• *Ghadiali's Spectro-Chrome*—This looks like something out of Buck Rogers. It's a box with colored lights. Green cures arthritis. Blue cures lung diseases. All you do is shine the appropriate light on the patient.

• *The Thermo-Magno-Ray Health Applicator*—It looks like a stainless steel bowl. You wear it on your head "to stimulate white blood cells to fight disease."

These and similar devices at the museum have one thing in common, Dr. Brodeur said: THEY'RE ALL WORTHLESS.

Horrible Effects of Quack Cures

Nine out of ten people with arthritis, or twenty-eight million people, have tried at least one worthless quack remedy. The remedies include burying oneself in cow manure, bathing joints in kerosene or whiskey, sitting in uranium mines for hours on end to absorb supposedly helpful rays, and rubbing aching joints with motor oil or ground-up rattails.

People who try these quack treatments aren't stupid—they're just desperate people trying desperate measures. Here are some of their stories.

• In southern California a man came close to dying after treatment in a Mexican clinic that left him horribly crippled and with badly damaged kidneys. In 1968, the man went to a Mexicali, Mexico, clinic where he received medicine prescribed by a doctor with all the usual diplomas on the walls of his office. The California man took the medicine for six months and wound up in the hospital, suffering intense pain all over his body.

"To my horror, I learned that this medicine was actually very high doses of cortisone," the man said. "What this quack treatment was doing was burning up my internal organs. I was hurting everywhere—the most excruciating pain I have ever experienced."

After that, he was left so badly crippled that he could never work again. He has had surgery to replace both knee joints, and his kidneys are so damaged he may have to be placed on a dialysis machine.

• A woman from New York City lost her hair and suffered severe hemorrhaging after taking a hazardous drug called *Liefcort.*

The woman traveled to Canada when she heard about a new drug called Liefcort. But she didn't know it contained hormones and dangerous steroids that subsequently wreaked havoc with her health.

"Horribly, a couple of weeks went by and I began hemorrhaging from the vagina and really began getting bloated. And then my hair began to come out in great big clumps. After the Liefcort treatment I had to have total hip surgery—and I learned that one of the side effects of Liefcort is bone problems. So it's likely that Liefcort caused my hip problem, not arthritis."

Liefcort has not been approved by the Food and Drug Administration for obvious reasons, but unfortunately it has been used by doctors in other countries.

Yet another terrifying story of quack treatments in arthritis involved the story of a victim who died while following a fad diet. Earlier, she had tried another idea—she danced naked under an oak tree during a full moon.

DMSO: Not a Wonder Drug

An example of the misleading and dangerous effects of the publicity surrounding an illegitimate treatment is the case of DMSO, a drug that is used by some as a liniment on the skin to help arthritis symptoms.

Although the Food and Drug Administration hasn't approved DMSO for use in arthritis treatment, sufferers across the country are using it.

Besides a possible reaction with Clinoril, the evidence is "rock hard" that DMSO also interferes with the ulcer drug *Tagamet* and the tranquilizer *Thorazine,* according to Dr. Peter Utsinger of the Germantown Hospital in Philadelphia.

DMSO is sold to the public as a solvent in many stores. Yet people use it as a liniment "because it has some pain-killing effects," says Dr. McDuffie of the Arthritis Foundation. But, he cautions, it is of no proven value for any form of arthritis.

Don't suffer needlessly while wasting your money. Go see a legitimate doctor who can put you on a program to help you lead a useful, productive, and happy life.

CHAPTER XII

Your Best Hope

IF YOU HAVE ARTHRITIS YOU ARE YOUR OWN BEST hope. All the medication, exercise, rest, tension relievers, self-help gadgets, and practical advice of fellow sufferers won't do a thing for you if you don't help yourself. Helping yourself means following the treatment program your doctor has devised for you; making an effort to try new ways to make your chores easier; talking with your family when you are angry or frustrated; not cheating on your exercises; and teaching someone how to be a real friend. This book is filled to overflowing with ideas that can help you. Use them. Experiment a little. Get your husband or children, friends or neighbors to help you. All the good advice and thoughtful tips won't help if you don't use them. So go ahead and get the most you can out of life—you deserve it.

With this in mind, we thought we might help you take a first step. Often the biggest problem in beginning is where to begin. Well, don't worry. We have decided that the best way to *end* our exploration of arthritis was to offer you a hand as you *begin* to live—to really *live*—with arthritis. Here are the twenty best steps to take to deal with the symptoms of arthritis. It's a quick rundown of practical and important ways to get relief, and was developed in conjunction with the Arthritis Foundation. Take these few pages and commit them to memory, or tack them to the wall in your kitchen. They are your reminder that you can't win the battle with arthritis, if you don't fight the war.

1. Plan your day with the proper balance of rest and activity. You need more rest than a person without arthritis. Most physicians recommend ten to twelve hours of rest for each twenty-four-hour period, divided between actual nighttime sleep and short periods of lying down or napping during the day.

When specific joints are inflamed, they often need special rest. Your therapist may recommend a resting splint to reduce stress on the joint.

2. Help yourself. It's not enough to go to the doctor or therapist and listen to what they say. Do things on your own at home—take your medication as prescribed and do your exercises.

3. Don't be afraid to ask questions. At home or in the hospital, a person has the right to ask about their health problems. Make sure you understand the words used, and don't hesitate to ask for a clearer explanation if needed.

4. Write down questions as you think of them, and show the list to your doctor or health-care professional when you see them.

5. Ask for written instructions regarding medications, exercise, or any procedure—it's too easy to forget.

6. Take a family member or friend when you visit your health-care professional. There will always be bits

of information that you or your doctor may fail to write down that your companion will remember. And after hearing your doctor's advice, a companion will be able to help you stick to the instructions.

7. Keep health records—a notebook or diary. It should contain what you've learned about your disease and what you're doing at home to care for yourself. Take it with you when you visit your doctor so you can answer his or her questions more accurately.

8. Practice energy conservation. Take breaks between tasks and don't feel that you have to complete big jobs all at once. Do what is most important, plan ahead, get help when you need it, and stop and rest before you become overly tired.

9. Remember that even when you have a painful arthritis flare-up, it's essential that you perform exercises prescribed by your doctor. Even though pain is usually made worse by any movement of the inflamed joint, you still must exercise it. If you don't move painful joints, they can quickly become stiff. If you don't regularly warm up or move your joints, the situation gets worse, leading to loss of motion, weakness, loss of function, and more pain.

10. Take your aspirin or anti-inflammatory medication an hour before you get out of bed in the morning. The night before, put your medication, a glass of water and a few crackers on your night table. Wake up an hour before you have to get up, then eat the crackers and take the pills. Having something to eat with the pills cuts the possibility of irritating an empty stomach.

11. Practice the "sandwich method" of taking medication—unless your doctor directs you otherwise. Eat a little food, take your medication, then eat a little more food. This will help protect the stomach.

12. Take a warm shower or bath immediately after you get up. In all cases, warm tap water should be sufficient to provide relief.

13. Do your limbering-up exercises after you shower or bathe, while you still feel warm.

14. Wear warm, adequate clothing in cold weather. Some people find that knitted woolen pullover cuffs on painful joints, especially the knees, ankles, and elbows, are helpful in keeping the joints warm in cold weather.

15. Try contrast baths to relieve painful flare-ups. For many people with arthritis, an effective approach is alternating warm and cold water applications, a process called contrast baths. It is most useful for a hand or foot which can be dipped in a large pot filled with water. Use a thermometer to check the water temperature.

Fill one container with 110-degree water, and fill another with 65-degree water. Put your hand or feet in the warm water for three minutes, then in the cold water for one minute. Repeat the process two more times, then go back to the warm bath for another three minutes.

16. Don't overdo heat or cold treatments. The maximum benefit from applying devices which will either heat or cool inflamed or stiff joints is achieved in twenty minutes.

Longer use of such devices as electric heating pads, hot packs or cold packs will not help the aching joint and could cause burns or skin damage.

17. Learn to respect pain—and know when it's a signal to stop what you are doing. A good general rule is that if an activity causes a joint to become painful—and the pain lingers for more than a few hours—it is harmful.

18. Maintain good basic nutrition. A normal, well-balanced, nourishing diet with adequate portions and good variety, three times a day—that's what you need.

Ignore advocates of special diets to combat arthritis. There has been no diet which has been proven scientifically to change the basic course of arthritis, or to cure it.

Keeping your weight under control is important because excessive weight produces added stress on joints.

19. Make your recreation fit your needs. Physically active sports, such as running, racquetball, or tennis, make severe demands on your joints and should not be engaged in until you have asked your physician.

Swimming can be a great way to exercise and not stress your joints. If card games or playing a musical instrument is your choice, remember to move around regularly to prevent stiffness.

Recreation can help you reduce mental stress, which is helpful when you are forced by arthritis to make major life-style changes.

20. Discuss your disease with your employer if it threatens your ability to keep working at your usual pace. Adjustments may have to be made on the job, so help your employer understand your condition. You may be able to continue on with your job as usual, or with a few changes such as rest breaks, relocation of itcms in your work space, a special chair, a modification of some tool, etc. Said Dr. McDuffie: "Your state department of vocational rehabilitation can offer advice to you and your employer on job modification—as well as possibly sharing expenses involved."

* * *

You can get a copy of the Arthritis Foundation's booklet, "Overcoming Rheumatoid Arthritis, What You Can Do Yourself"—on which this chapter was based. Although the booklet is specifically designed to help persons with rheumatoid arthritis overcome their pain, the tips included in this chapter will help people with arthritis.

APPENDIX

State and Local Chapters of the Arthritis Foundation

Founded in 1948, the Arthritis Foundation is the only national, voluntarily supported organization working to solve the problems and mysteries of arthritis in all its forms.

State and community chapters support local scientific investigation and clinical research centers. The chapters also support educational programs to provide people with arthritis with as much help as possible in improving the quality of their lives in spite of having arthritis.

For information, contact your local chapter.

Alabama

Alabama Chapter
13 Office Park Circle
Birmingham, AL 35223

South Alabama Chapter
304 Little Flower Avenue
Mobile, AL 36606

Arizona

Central Arizona Chapter
2102 West Indian School Road
Suite 9
Phoenix, AZ 85015

Southern Arizona Chapter
3813 East Second Street
Tucson, AZ 85716

Arkansas

Arkansas Chapter
6213 Lee Avenue
Little Rock, AK 72205

California

Northeastern California Chapter
1722 "J" Street
Sacramento, CA 95814

Northern California Chapter
185 Berry Street
Building 3, Suite 363
San Francisco, CA 94107

San Diego Area Chapter
6154 Mission Gorge Road
San Diego, CA 92120

Southern California Chapter
5311 Wilshire Boulevard
Los Angeles, CA 90010

Colorado

Rocky Mountain Chapter
243 Columbine Street
Denver, CO 80206

Connecticut

Connecticut Chapter
929 Silas Deane Highway
Wethersfield, CT 06109

Delaware

Delaware Chapter
234 Philadelphia Pike
Wilmington, DE 19809

District of Columbia

Metropolitan Washington Chapter
2424 Pennsylvania Avenue
Washington, DC 20037

Florida

Florida Chapter
3205 Manatee Avenue West
Bradenton, FL 33505

Georgia

Georgia Chapter
2799 Delk Road, S.E.
Marietta, GA 30067

Metropolitan Branch
C&S Northeast Center
2059 Collridge Road
Tucker, GA 30084

Hawaii

Hawaii Chapter
200 North Vineyard
Honolulu, HI 96817

Idaho

Idaho Chapter
700 Robbins Road
Boise, Idaho 83702

Illinois

Central Illinois Chapter
Allied Agencies Center
320 East Armstrong Avenue
Peoria, IL 61603

Illinois Chapter
79 West Monroe
Chicago, IL 60603

Indiana

Indiana Chapter
1010 East 86th Street
Indianapolis, IN 46240

Iowa

Iowa Chapter
1501 Ingersoll Avenue
Des Moines, IA 50309

Kansas

Kansas Chapter
1602 East Waterman
Wichita, KA 67211

Kentucky

Kentucky Chapter
1381 Bardstown Road
Louisville, KY 40204

Louisiana

Louisiana Chapter
4700 Dryades
New Orleans, LA 70115

Maine

Maine Chapter
37 Mill Street
Brunswick, ME 04011

Maryland

Maryland Chapter
12 West 25th Street
Baltimore, MD 21218

Massachusetts

Massachusetts Chapter
59 Temple Place
Boston, MA 02111

Michigan

Michigan Chapter
23400 Michigan
Suite 605
Dearborn, MI 48124

Minnesota

Minnesota Chapter
122 West Franklin
Minneapolis, MN 55404

Mississippi

Mississippi Chapter
6055 Ridgewood Road
Jackson, MS 39211

Missouri

Eastern Missouri Chapter
4144 Lindell Boulevard
St. Louis, MO 63108

Greater Kansas City Chapter
8301 State Line Road
Kansas City, MO 64114

Montana

Montana Chapter
P.O. Box 20994
Billings, MT 59104

Nebraska

Nebraska Chapter
120 North 69th Street
Omaha, NE 68132

Nevada

Nevada Division
2700 State Street
Las Vegas, NV 89104

New Hampshire

New Hampshire Chapter
P.O. Box 369
Concord, NH 03301

New Jersey

New Jersey Chapter
15 Prospect Street
Colonia, NJ 07067

New Mexico

New Mexico Chapter
5112 Grand Avenue N.E.
Albuquerque, NM 87108

New York

Central New York Chapter
505 East Fayette Street
Syracuse, NY 13212

Genesee Valley Chapter
973 East Avenue
Rochester, NY 14607

Long Island Division
501 Walt Whitman Road
Melville, NY 11747

New York Chapter
115 East 18th Street
New York, NY 10003

Northeastern New York Chapter
1237 Central Avenue
Albany, NY 12205

Western New York Chapter
4556 Baily Avenue
Buffalo, NY 14226

North Carolina

North Carolina Chapter
P.O. Box 2505
Durham, NC 27705

North Dakota

Dakota Chapter
1402 N. 39th Street
Fargo, ND 58102

Ohio

Akron Area Chapter
326 Locust Street
Akron, OH 44302

Central Ohio Chapter
2501 North Star Road
Columbus, OH 43221

Northeastern Ohio Chapter
11416 Bellflower Road
Cleveland, OH 44106

Northwestern Ohio Chapter
4447 Talmadge Road
Toledo, OH 43623

Southwestern Ohio Chapter
2400 Reading Road
Cincinnati, OH 45202

Oklahoma

Eastern Oklahoma Chapter
2615-D South Memorial
Tulsa, OK 74129

Oklahoma Chapter
3313 Classen Boulevard
Oklahoma City, OK 73118

Oregon

Oregon Chapter
2330 North West Flanders
Portland, OR 92207

Pennsylvania

Central Pennsylvania Chapter
P.O. Box 668
Camp Hill, PA 17011

Eastern Pennsylvania Chapter
311 South Juniper Street
Philadelphia, PA 19107

Western Pennsylvania Chapter
2201 Clark Building
Pittsburgh, PA 15222

Rhode Island

Rhode Island Chapter
850 Waterman Avenue
East Providence, RI 02914

South Carolina

South Carolina Chapter
3008 Millwood Avenue
Columbia, SC 29205

Tennessee

Middle East Tennessee Chapter
1719 West End Building
Nashville, TN 37203

West Tennessee Chapter
2600 Poplar Avenue
Memphis, TN 38112

Texas

North Texas Chapter
5415 Maple Avenue
Dallas, TX 75235

Northwest Texas Chapter
3145 McCart Avenue
Fort Worth, TX 76110

South Central Texas
Chapter
503 South Main Street
San Antonio, TX 78204

Texas Gulf Coast Chapter
9099-A Katy Freeway
Houston, TX 77024

West Texas Chapter
1926 34th Street
Lubbock, TX 79401

Utah

Utah Chapter
Graystone Plaza
1174 East 2700 South
Salt Lake City, UT 84106

Vermont

Vermont Chapter
215 College Street
Burlington, VT 05401

Virginia

Peninsula Branch
12388 Warwick Boulevard
Newport News, VA 23606

Virginia Chapter
P.O. Box 6772
Richmond, VA 23230

Washington

Western Washington
Chapter
726 Broadway
Seattle, WA 98122

West Virginia

West Virginia Chapter
P.O. Box 8473
South Charleston,
WV 25303

Wisconsin

Wisconsin Chapter
1442 North Farewell
Avenue
Milwaukee, WI 53202